Oedipus and Beyond

JAY GREENBERG

Oedipus and Beyond
A CLINICAL THEORY

HARVARD UNIVERSITY PRESS
CAMBRIDGE, MASSACHUSETTS
LONDON, ENGLAND
1991

This book is printed on acid-free paper, and its binding
materials have been chosen for strength and durability.

Library of Congress Cataloging-in-Publication Data

Greenberg, Jay R.
  Oedipus and beyond : a clinical theory / Jay Greenberg.
    p.   cm.
  Includes bibliographical references and index.
  ISBN 0–674–63090-4 (alk. paper)
  1. Psychoanalysis.   2. Motivation (Psychology)   3. Oedipus
complex.   4. Instinct.   5. Freud, Sigmund, 1856–1939.   I. Title.
  [DNLM: 1. Freudian Theory.   2. Models, Psychological.
3. Oedipus Complex. WM 460 G79850]
RC506.G74   1991
150.19′52—dc20
DNLM/DLC
for Library of Congress   91–7078
                                                              CIP

For Olga

Preface

THIS BOOK began as it will end, with some unfinished business. In *Object Relations in Psychoanalytic Theory* Stephen Mitchell and I distinguished between two major psychoanalytic models: a drive model, developed by Freud and his followers within the classical tradition; and a relational model, based on the radical rejection of drive in favor of a view that all motivation unfolds from our personal experience of exchanges with others. We argued that the two models are incompatible, that they reflect ancient and irreconcilably alternative visions of the human condition. We suggested that the existence of differences between the models—holding out the promise of continuing debate among adherents of each—is healthy both for clinical practice and for psychoanalysis as a discipline.

I still believe that the two models are incompatible and that diversity is our best guarantee of vitality. But the conviction generates its own vexing questions, highlighted by my experience as a clinical psychoanalyst. It seems, to me at least, that the psychoanalytic situation is fundamentally and inexorably social; after decades of theoretical acrobatics to the contrary, we must acknowledge that the mutual influence of analyst and analysand is constant in any treatment. At the same time, doing analysis reveals how profoundly personal and, when all is said and done, how private our experience is. The two thoughts, taken together, define a paradox at the very core of our clinical work.

The paradox illuminates both the power and the limits of each psychoanalytic model. Freud's vision of the innate, presocial, even unspeakable passions that move us captures the uniquely individual world within which each of us lives. Yet it cannot account well enough for the relentless effects of interpersonal living. Theorists operating within the relational

model have exquisitely portrayed the way experience is shaped by social influence. But the premises of their model make it difficult to see the decisive ways in which people shape interpersonal experience itself; the model is weak at conceptualizing what each of us "brings to the party."

So I begin with the unfinished business not of combining the models but of trying to extract from each of them what fits best with my understanding of people generally and of my patients in particular. The project has led me deeply into the structure—into the metapsychology, to use a currently unfashionable term—of each model. In the Introduction and Chapters 1 through 4, and again in Chapter 6, I explore some fundamental theoretical constructs, always with a view toward clarifying how taking a particular position will affect the clinical enterprise. I review both drive and structural concepts, because I believe that our views on each have decisive implications for how we set up the psychoanalytic situation and for our interpretive posture.

After discussing the evolution and current status of different approaches, I take my own positions on some of the central issues that I have identified; this is the focus of Chapters 5, 7, and 8. There I generate some new unfinished business: a new model that reflects the kind of work I do. But I don't think of what I have come up with as a final answer, or even as an answer at all. Theory is not a solution; it is a tool. When we theorize we apply our assumptions, drawn from some place or other (psychoanalytic books, other writings, life as we have lived it), to what we see clinically. If the assumptions are generative, they will shape what we observe; but they themselves will be altered by the observations. The function of theory is to provide a framework for observations, and eventually to yield. This was the fate of Freud's various models throughout his lifetime. The seduction theory gave way, but without it Freud might never have arrived at his appreciation of the importance of psychic reality. The same can be said of the topographic model, the first anxiety theory, and the first dual-instinct theory. Ultimately all fruitful theory is self-extinguishing because it generates the data that lead to its demise.

I have titled Part III of the book "Technical Implications," and there I discuss how I go about establishing a useful analytic ambience and also how I think about transference and countertransference. Although I refer to "implications" for technique, the relationship between my theoretical conceptualizing and my clinical style is circular. This was driven home to me forcefully as I was writing the book; frequently I noticed unexpected parallels between my most abstract musings and what I do on a daily basis

with my patients. Catching on to this relationship has been exciting; my hope for the book is that it will encourage others to discover unexpected connections among various facets of their experience as psychoanalysts and psychotherapists.

I owe many debts of gratitude for encouragement, support, and help that have been extended to me during my work on the book. Several chapters were written in response to invitations to share my ideas with various organizations. These include the William Alanson White Psychoanalytic Society, the Washington D.C. Psychoanalytic Society, the Southern California Psychoanalytic Society, the Association for Psychoanalytic Medicine, the Menninger Foundation, the Topeka Psychoanalytic Institute, and the Tufts University School of Medicine. Some of my ideas have appeared in preliminary form in *Contemporary Psychoanalysis, Psychoanalytic Dialogues, Psychoanalytic Inquiry,* and *Psychoanalytic Psychology,* and I thank the publishers of those journals for their many courtesies: the William Alanson White Institute, the Analytic Press, and Lawrence Erlbaum Associates.

I am particularly grateful for and optimistic about the interest in psychoanalysis that has been generated around the United States by local chapters of the Division of Psychoanalysis, American Psychological Association. Some groups have honored me by asking me to speak, and I want to thank those in Denver, Boston, San Francisco, Chicago, Dallas, Miami, and New Haven. Several chapters have spawned training institutes, each of which is characterized by a commitment to psychoanalysis and an openness to new ideas that augur well for the future of our discipline. I have gained a great deal from my affiliations with the Colorado Center for Psychoanalytic Studies, the Massachusetts Institute for Psychoanalysis, and the Psychoanalytic Institute of Northern California.

A number of people have been helpful and supportive as I worked on the book. Milton Eber, Kenneth Eisold, Jay Kwawer, and Harold Sampson read all or part of the manuscript and had important and encouraging things to say. A study group in Oklahoma City led by Martha Jo Shaw read an early draft book and were kind enough to invite me to discuss the work in progress in a seminar; their responses stimulated and heartened me.

Four analysts have been particularly generous with their time and effort in going over the manuscript. Philip Bromberg, Merton Gill, Stephen Mitchell, and Charles Spezzano read everything carefully, challenged a

great deal, and argued their points well. While each found much to disagree with, I emerged from our exchanges feeling sustained by their support and friendship. They have influenced both my feelings about the venture and the eventual product itself.

Finally, and above all, there are my wife and children. My daughters Carla and Melissa have put up with a lot throughout my work on the book. They have been patient and understanding, often beyond their years. More than that, their lives touch everything in this book (and in their father) in ways they won't fully understand for a long time to come. My wife, Olga Cheselka, has sustained and encouraged me through all the ups and downs of a long, difficult project. Frequently I gave her drafts to read even before I dared look at them myself. Her unwavering support emboldened me to go on; without her, the book simply would not be.

Contents

Oedipus and Beyond

Introduction: Toward a New Oedipus Complex

PSYCHOANALYSIS, a century after its origin in the scientific and therapeutic ambitions of Sigmund Freud, remains in the shadow of its creator. Freud's monumental genius and charismatic leadership generated not only an intellectual discipline but a movement with deep personal ties to its founder. Today his presence remains as compelling to those who reject his particular psychoanalytic vision as to those who accept it. All analysts begin with and react to Freud; we are in a constant dialectic with him. "Freudianism" is both partisan and conceptual; it is an inevitable if sometimes subliminal presence in almost every psychoanalytic debate.

Freud's brilliance as thinker and leader was vital in establishing a uniquely problematic field of inquiry. Psychoanalysis is, by definition, the study of what people don't want to know about: Freud's creation forces us to confront the motivated gaps in self-understanding brought about by the disavowal of painful experience. Our most poignant desires, our deepest fears about ourselves, the most carefully guarded secrets of family life—these are the everyday stuff of analytic thinking. Without Freud's supreme self-confidence, and without his followers' (and critics') idealization of him, it is unlikely that these could have become the focus of organized study.

It is no accident that psychoanalysis was invented by a man capable of working with virtually no institutional support for more than a decade. An approach to human nature and its pathology as bold as Freud's could not have evolved in any other way. Nor have the obstacles to a truly psychoanalytic vision disappeared. Though over the years a range of Freudian and neo-Freudian concepts has been absorbed into the intellectual life of our culture, maintaining a deeply felt analytic attitude remains difficult

today. Not only the content (still and always what is disavowed) but the style of analytic thinking is out of step with contemporary standards. Our technologically oriented society values the tangible, the certain, and the fast-paced; analysts live with the ineffable, the complex, and the painstaking. The disjunction encourages continuing dependence on a relationship with a strong founder and with the inheritors of his legacy, embodied in the institutions that psychoanalysis has created.

But psychoanalysis has paid a heavy price for institutionalizing its creator. An analyst's declared relation to Freud continues to determine his or her place in the professional community; academic opportunity and even economic well-being depend on these commitments. Because of this, interpretations of Freud are tinged by political intent. One need only examine the torturous attempts of some contemporary theorists to tie their views to what Freud said or to what he didn't say but "really meant." Or the equally torturous efforts of others to build theory through a confrontation with Freud that often depends on similarly strained interpretations of his writings. Both his advocates and his critics took the lifelong labors of a genius struggling to grasp the human condition and made it into doctrine. As a result, many of Freud's most original and challenging ideas lost their vitality. When probing became scripture, when hypothesis became directive, conceptual development was sacrificed to fealty and rebellion. All this has had a seriously inhibiting effect on the development of psychoanalytic theory.

Freud's psychoanalytic theory of motivation has been especially affected by the changed intellectual climate. The theory is particularly important for clinical practice because it addresses the "why" of behavior and experience, and so forms the basis of the listening analyst's interpretive armamentarium. By almost all accounts, psychoanalysis works through some version of making the unconscious conscious; deepening analysands' experience of their own motivations is central to this expansion of self-awareness.

Psychoanalysis began as a radical theory of motivation: Freud claimed to cure the incurable by explaining the inexplicable. Over the course of several decades he laid down four motivational principles, each of which powerfully challenged conventional wisdom. First, all mental activity is motivated (the principle of psychic determinism). Second, motives can and generally do operate outside of conscious awareness. Third, no mental event has a unitary motive; human experience is inevitably the product of conflicting tendencies and compromises. Finally, all motivation is traceable

ultimately to the operation of biologically rooted, phylogenetically determined sexual and destructive needs. These needs are experienced as urges or impulses and reflect the working of elementary human instincts, or drives.

Each of Freud's principles implies a vision of human nature that defies valued aspects of our self-concept. Psychic determinism undermines convenient disavowal of personal meaning; the challenge becomes palpable in our reluctance to explore dreams or Freudian slips. Unconscious motivation, as Freud often noted, weakens the sense of ourselves as master in our own house; no longer can we insist that reason alone guides our actions. Conflict theory drives home both the complexity and the unavoidable incompatibility of "natural" human goals. Neither uncomplicated altruism nor simple self-interest adequately explains behavior. The libido/aggression theory, binding our inner nature—not only our outer appearance—to a Darwinian past, reminds us that "human" does not necessarily mean "higher" and that the nobility with which we tend to clothe our goals is illusory or even self-deceptive.

Although each is radical, Freud's four motivational principles have notably different implications. It should be possible for the contemporary analyst to address each individually, to accept what accords with his clinical experience and to reject what does not. Unfortunately, the politicization of Freud has made this extremely difficult. Psychoanalytic theory has become a proprietary commodity, and "Freudian" propositions are treated as a package, accepted or rejected in its entirety. The special problem of the theory of motivation is that all four principles have become condensed into the libido/aggression concept. Thus one rarely sees references to "conflict" that do not imply that sexual or destructive impulses are parties to the conflict. Analysts who base their interpretive systems on conflict theory assume the centrality of these impulses. Even more strikingly, those who wish to get away from libido/aggression theory, evidently accepting the package, tend to talk about people as nonconflictual or preconflictual. Similarly, many analysts equate the unconscious itself with warded-off sexual and aggressive impulses; they believe that the revisionists who have rejected Freud's dual-instinct theory must also have rejected the notion of a dynamic unconscious (see Curtis, 1985).

At its extreme, the proprietary treatment of Freud has led to the condensation of two distantly related ideas: the hypothesis that all behavior is motivated and the hypothesis that all motivation is a transformation of innate sexual and aggressive impulses. The confusion originates in Freud's

own words. In his most important definition of drive *(Trieb)*, it is "a demand made upon the mind for work" (1905a, p. 168; 1915a, p. 122) and "the ultimate cause of all activity" (1940, p. 148). The train of thought runs as follows: To talk about motive is to talk about drive; to talk about drive is to talk about Freud's particular dual-instinct theory; therefore to talk about motive—especially the unconscious motive that is of greatest interest clinically—is to talk about sexuality and aggression.

Let me demonstrate how this conceptual condensation works. Hans Loewald, in taking issue with the concept of primarily autonomous ego apparatuses, argues that "libidinal-aggressive elements remain ingredients of perception and memory . . . and constitute the unconscious motivational aspect of the latter" (1977, pp. 209–210). This is an empirical assertion: Loewald holds that instinctual aims are never entirely stripped from cognitive operations, as Heinz Hartmann and his followers claimed they could be. He chooses not to address the problem of whether these functions can, in principle, operate in the service of motives derived neither from libido nor from aggression. But some authors go further: if a mental act is not fueled by libido and aggression, they claim, it is not motivated at all. Ernst Kris (1956), for example, believes that we can reach a level of maturity at which objective self-observation—uncontaminated by motive—is possible. A comment by Morris Eagle takes this to its extreme, explicitly collapsing Freud's motivational principles: "the very concept of unconscious motives and the principle of universal motivational determinism are linked to a theory of instincts . . . Freud's psychic determinism *really* constitutes a claim that all behavior . . . reflects the operation of instinctual wishes constantly pressing for discharge" (1980, p. 340, my italics).

An adequate psychoanalytic theory must account for the motivational aspects of perception, memory, and objective self-observation. Every analyst knows that these activities are motivated, that they often serve unconscious aims, and that their operation is influenced by the conflicting goals they serve. Thus they are subject to three of Freud's four principles of motivation. But many analysts have found it impossible to bring these activities under the fourth principle; they cannot be explained simply as transformations of sexual or destructive impulses.

This widely acknowledged observation should constitute a strong argument for dropping the libido/aggression theory while retaining the principles of psychic determinism, unconscious motivation, and ubiquitous conflict. But, because Freud's four principles have been condensed

into a package, the expected challenge has not occurred. Loyalists, unwilling to yield the motivational centrality of sexuality and aggression, compartmentalized mental life, introducing the unwieldy and improbable concept of neutralization and the "miserly" (Erikson, 1962) notion of a conflict-free sphere. Critics, implicitly accepting the linkage, have felt it necessary to reject not only the dual-instinct theory but the centrality of conflict (Kohut, Guntrip) and even of motivational determinism itself (Gedo, 1979).

As a result of these strategies, the theoretical tail of psychoanalysis wags the dog. Hard-won insights, gained over decades of observation by thousands of observers, are treated as handmaidens to the Freudian drives. The unconscious and the central role of personal motivation have been sacrificed to libido theory. An original, complex, evolving vision of human nature shrivels, becoming something old and static. In much of this, psychoanalysis caricatures itself. Critics' mutually contradictory charges of pan-sexuality and naive environmentalism aptly characterize much of our theory, if not our clinical practice.

ONE OF the casualties of the politicization of drive theory has been the Oedipus complex. A richly textured clinical and theoretical construct, in much recent psychoanalytic debate the Oedipus complex is little more than a slogan. My purpose in the remainder of this chapter will be twofold. First, I will attempt to show how the Oedipus complex has fallen victim to the politically motivated conceptual condensation I have been describing. Second, I will introduce some considerations that may point the way to the development of a "new" Oedipus complex, one that accords more fully with clinical experience as it has been reported by many analysts over many years.

For Freud, the Oedipus complex was both the nodal event of normal development and the core conflict of the neuroses; the interplay of psychic forces in both mental health and psychopathology becomes comprehensible in its context. It is an extraordinary analytic invention, a framework for conceptualizing family dynamics and their residue in the psychic life of the child. But now the Oedipus complex is as much an institutional as a clinical/theoretical issue. Freud, always the protagonist of his own political battles, is partially responsible for this. In one of his formulations he called the Oedipus complex a "shibboleth" of psychoanalysis—a hallmark of true belief (1905a, p. 226n). Today an analyst's attitude toward the primacy of so-called "oedipal" as opposed to "preoedipal" dynamics re-

mains a key determinant of his place in the psychoanalytic community. This leads to a jockeying for lineage that obscures just how complex the Oedipus complex actually is. Shibboleths ought to be straightforward and simple; the Oedipus complex is elaborate and elusive. Even a fairly simple version of it contains a large number of related but logically independent propositions.

Ages Three to Six: A Phenomenology

I will begin by presenting a brief summary of the oedipal situation. It will quickly become clear that any such account represents an intricate array of observations, inferences, theoretical assumptions, and so on. Nowhere in psychoanalysis is it more difficult, as Hartmann, Kris, and Loewenstein remark, "to distinguish at which point theory ceases and observation begins" (1953, p. 120). But I will attempt to begin as nearly as possible with description, moving from there to putatively explanatory theoretical constructs.

The child (I refer to the young girl for economy of exposition and also to stress important elements of the Oedipus complex that are experienced similarly by both sexes) between approximately the ages of three and six indicates, in more or less verbalized fantasies, that she is involved in a new and striking way with her parents. She talks with increasing conviction of being a grown-up someday. When she gets bigger, she will replace her mother and marry her father, or she will marry somebody unmistakably (from the adults' perspective) like him. Plans for having babies of her own are discussed. The child spends a good deal of time thinking about growing; she fully intends to become as big and as strong as her parents. Potency and fertility become increasingly compelling.

The child's nonverbal behavior reflects a similar development. Her games take on a competitive and even combative cast. The child learns about winning and losing, and the outcome of games acquires a powerful new importance. She embraces victory and recoils from defeat, which previously were of little concern. She begins to act in a sexually suggestive way, inviting overt manipulation of her genitals as well as making less direct seductive overtures.

The child's fantasies of being or of becoming big, strong, and powerful are matched by an increasing sense of being excluded from her parents' relationship with each other. The four-year-old is likely to notice and object to the fact that her parents sleep together while she sleeps alone. Fre-

quently the child will interrupt her parents' privacy, giving clear indication that she resents it.

For the first time during this period, the state of the child's relationship with one parent strongly influences the state of her relationship with the other. Particularly intense affectionate feelings for one parent are likely to evoke intense rivalrous feelings for the other. The child's predominant attitude is one of affection toward the cross-sex parent and rivalry toward the same-sex parent, although this is certainly more variable than psychoanalytic theory would lead us to believe. The advent of triangulation does not simply reflect the child's relationships within the family. During this phase of her life she is also meeting new people outside the home, in school, and so on. For the first time she is developing relationships that are not brokered by her parents.

Triangulation is interesting and important because it heralds the child's more complex, textured experience of her life. Cause and effect now transcend the immediate environment as represented by the dyad; need and desire have an impact across temporal and spatial distance. There are new worlds to be mastered, and their various, often competing demands must be measured against one another.

The child begins to be aware of this; more and more, she gives the impression that she understands that important choices are to be made. She learns to weigh alternatives and to pursue what she wants vigorously. The child's new understanding and capabilities, along with her growth and ambitions and along with her awareness of exclusion from moments shared by her parents, contribute to an evolving sense of separateness; she reacts to this with both pride and frustration. The sense of separateness impresses outsiders. Frequently one notices the child engaged in an inner dialogue. Increasingly she appears self-contained.

It is apparent that the events of ages three to six make this a very special time in the child's life. They are so striking that they warrant definition as a unique phase in development: the passage from infancy to childhood. Extrapolating further, these years represent the gateway to successful adulthood. The events that occur are the keys to the development of psychic structure and mature relations with others.

Freud's Achievement

The changes that the child goes through as she emerges from infancy have always been felt keenly by every parent and noticed by observers. Freud's

genius was to create a narrative that gave these years a shape and to use it as part of a therapeutic inquiry into his patients' life histories. Because they are so crucial to normal development, it makes sense to assume that the events of ages three to six are essential components of the nuclear conflict in the neuroses. Freud argued that the presence of neurotic symptoms or neurotic-level character pathology required and could be explained only by some failure to resolve the problems of this developmental phase. From a clinical perspective, Freudian analysis became analysis of these problems. With this, Freud invented the Oedipus complex.

Two related characteristics of the Oedipus complex explain its utility as the focus of analytic inquiry. Both follow from the fact that oedipal experiences occur at a time when the child has achieved considerable ego development. First, the child is able to form and pursue structured, coherent goals and to do so with a relative, if often disavowed, sense of personal agency. Similarly, her increased cognitive maturity permits the formation of stable object representations and makes it possible for the child to encode both goals and representations as verbally accessible (though often repressed) memories. Second, the child's experience is now significantly determined by her fantasies—the imaginings about growing up, marrying, and having babies are commonplace examples. The emergence of triangulated relational experience plays a role in this development; inevitably the child imagines the effects of her actions on people who are not immediately present. Thus the centrality of the Oedipus complex implies an emphasis on the role of fantasy unfolding from within not only as a determinant of childhood experience but also as a force in the psychic reality of the adult analysand (see Arlow, 1980, 1985a).

Even attempting to describe the Oedipus complex simply leads us quickly to a vast range of human motives, affects, and capacities. The child I have portrayed is bound to feel, among other powerful emotions: wildly oscillating love, hate, and need directed toward the same person; loyalties torn between the two people most important to her; exclusion from what seems most desirable, along with its attendant self-contempt and jealousy; guilt over her ambitions and shame for her failures; new hope for the future; fear of retaliation from her rivals; and a dawning sense of herself as a separate individual with untold potential and intolerable limitations. All of these feelings have an important relation on the one hand to innate, spontaneously generated goals experienced as impulses and, on the other hand, to newly emerging imaginative and other cognitive capabilities.

These feelings emerge from a complex mix of internal wishes and inter-

personal exchanges. Although he believed that it is ubiquitous, occurring in all individuals regardless of familial or cultural circumstances and significantly determined by endogenous (phylogenetic and instinctual) forces, Freud did not think that the Oedipus complex was simply an intriguing post-toddler fantasy. The oedipal child, as she is increasingly (if not consciously) aware, is the object as well as the subject of what goes on. Freud made several references to the causal role of interpersonal transactions in the onset of the Oedipus complex. In his study of Leonardo da Vinci (1910a) and in the Wolf Man case history (1918), he suggests that the child's personal experience of the oedipal years will be significantly affected by parental attitudes, both conscious and unconscious. In his strongest formulation, he argues that the child's incestuous object choice usually follows some "indication from its parents, whose affection bears the clearest characteristics of a sexual activity . . . As a rule a father prefers his daughter and a mother her son; the child reacts to this by wishing, if he is a son, to take his father's place, and, if she is a daughter, her mother's" (1910b, p. 47). These clinical observations so impressed Freud that, according to Rapaport, the Oedipus complex stands as a testament to his belief in the importance of the "social determination of behavior" (1959, p. 63).

Interpersonal factors determine oedipal dangers more directly than they affect oedipal wishes. The clearest example is the boy's fear of physical retaliation by his rivalrous father. In the prototypical case history of Little Hans, Freud tells us that the castration fear expressed through Hans's phobia was "realistic," based on the child's best assessment of the dangers lurking beneath the superficial serenity of family life (1926, p. 108). Hartmann and Kris are even more explicit. Castration fears, they write, are derived at least in part from "the veiled aggression of the adult against the child" (1945, p. 18). Thus the fully experienced Oedipus complex is a good example of the workings of what Freud called the "complemental series" (1916/1917, p. 347). It is constructed out of the interplay of internally derived motives and the external circumstances within which those motives are expressed.

When we include family dynamics in our observational field, the intricacy of the Oedipus complex looks even more impressive. The child has, certainly from her own perspective, been seduced, rejected, threatened, and humiliated—all by those whom she loves and who love her the most. At the same time, she is under increasing pressure to be socialized, to behave in a modulated way that is acceptable within the culture of which

she is a part. And she begins to see herself and to be treated by others not as a grown-up, certainly, but as a somewhat individuated participant in the social order (see Loewald, 1978), as a person among other people. The Oedipus complex marks the end of infancy, for better and for worse.

If what I have been discussing seems to describe the process of becoming human, condensed into what Peter Gay has called a "portentous domestic encounter" (1985, p. 95), it is because this is how I read the Oedipus complex. Seen this way, the oedipal story sums up the child's development first toward involvement in and then toward separation from the family. The Oedipus complex concentrates the deepest passions of family life and brings them to a head. For Gay, it expresses "man's fundamental and ineradicable ambivalence—the often unresolvable coexistence of love and hatred" (1985, p. 95).

Growing up requires coming to terms with this ambivalence. We must all find a way to pursue our personal ambitions, to live with other people, and to create our own families. These achievements depend upon the partial renunciation of oedipal wishes, an occurrence that Freud thought was necessary largely because of the dangers (typically focused on banishment and physical punishment) that the child comes to associate with them. Renunciation is so difficult that a special mental operation develops to make it possible: the oedipal conflicts succumb to repression, and the associated wishes and fears move off the center stage of consciousness. Leaving behind the associated fantasies is assumed to be painful for the child; it involves both acceptance of her own limits as a person and the loss of a powerful and exciting, if largely illusory, object relationship.

But Freud believed that there is ample, if not so immediately gratifying, compensation for the loss. Ego and especially superego identifications are achieved, he said, and these both depend upon and facilitate the postponement of goals that had seemed urgent and the pursuit of more realistic goals. The increased consolidation of psychic structure permits the child to experience a variety of wishes in the context of an ongoing sense of well-being and self-esteem. Although most analysts follow Freud and stress the forbidden when they discuss oedipal resolution, the consolidation of what is permitted is at least equally important. Thus the child is able to establish and maintain permanent and satisfying aim-inhibited relationships within the family. Further, despite having suffered an object loss, she has gained the freedom to pursue pleasure with appropriate extrafamilial objects. In an important sense, the passing of the Oedipus complex reflects, in terms of Freud's early model, an account of human development similar to that suggested much later by Margaret Mahler in her

theory of the separation-individuation process. As the gateway to permissible relationships with available objects, it represents separation. As the key event in psychic structure formation, it is the pathway to individuation.

FOR A while now it has been fashionable in some psychoanalytic circles to move the Oedipus complex into the wings. The argument is that many if not most patients' development has been arrested at an earlier stage. So-called preoedipal patients are thought to be struggling with different concerns; their problems must be conceptualized in alternative dynamic terms, and they must be treated differently. But the Oedipus complex cannot be disposed of so easily. What distinguishes the oedipal from the preoedipal patient? From the perspective of the Oedipus complex as a psychoanalytic concept, what are the clinical sensibilities here? I would suggest that the core of the Oedipus complex contains three propositions with implications for how people are to be approached clinically. First, patients are to be understood as the active agents of their experience; second, fantasy plays a central role in the formation of experience, and fantasy itself is significantly shaped by the person's inner needs; third, intrapsychic conflict is an inevitable aspect of motive and feeling. Consider the similarity to the first three of the broad motivational principles mentioned at the beginning: I am suggesting that the Oedipus complex first constructs a developmental event and then interprets that event in terms of these principles. Let me summarize the thinking behind my formulation of each proposition.

The role of agency. The key event along the path to mature mental health is the establishment and resolution of an intrafamilial relationship in which the child experiences particularly intense, potentially destabilizing, feelings for both parents. This central crisis does not occur until the child is about three or four years old, so considerable psychic development has already taken place. The older child can be credited with forming structured, coherent, clinically interpretable goals; her motives have a discernible and characteristic direction. Therefore a certain amount of intentionality is assumed; the child, and later the patient, is presumed to be the agent of her actions. This is implicit in the frequently asserted technical rule that experience must be at least potentially verbalizable to be clinically reliable. Especially from the perspective of clinical psychoanalysis, earlier experience is not necessarily more basic or more influential in the formation of personality.

The role of fantasy. Also as a result of understanding the key developmen-

tal crisis as emerging when there is relatively sophisticated mental equipment, the experience is assumed to occur when the child has achieved considerable imaginative capacity. Thus the original relationships with family members are significantly determined by the nature of the child's fantasies. Further, as the vicissitudes of the original crisis continue to influence psychic experience throughout life, the effect is exerted through the persistence of the early fantasies. The oedipal fantasies—both those that contributed to the original domestic drama and their elaborations in later life—are substantially shaped by the individual's endogenously generated need. These needs grow out of the child's developmental requirements. Specifying the nature of these needs is an important function of psychoanalytic theory.

The role of conflict. The child's, and later the adult's, various passionate desires give rise to powerfully conflicting motives. These include, at the least: ambivalent conflicts, in which the individual directs contradictory feelings toward one person; and conflicts of loyalty, in which attachments to and interests in the parents must be balanced against each other. These conflicts evoke intense affects, which last throughout life. Guilt is the child's principal negative reaction to her new motives and their attendant object relations, while shame and jealousy are also felt to a significant degree. Although positive affects are relatively neglected in theoretical formulations, it is important to keep in mind that the child also feels pride in her new capacities, ambition to use them in a variety of ways, and excitement about her prospects for the future.

Although I am suggesting that a full formulation of the Oedipus complex includes propositions relating to personal agency, the role of fantasies that are shaped by inner needs, and the ubiquity of intrapsychic conflict, note that the three propositions are logically independent. Each is debatable in its own right, and an analyst's position on each one plays an important role in defining his particular psychoanalytic vision, his way of understanding and working with patients.

The Oedipal Shibboleth

Where in all this is anything that might be called a shibboleth of true belief in psychoanalysis? Just what in the oedipal drama distinguishes true believer from heretic? Leo Rangell has asserted that a properly conducted analysis *always* reveals oedipal material at the core of neurotic processes. If such material is not uncovered, this is simply evidence that the technique

employed was faulty and superficial (Rangell, 1954, 1982). But what does that mean? What does the Freudian analyst discover when he "finds" his patient's Oedipus complex? Does he find agency, fantasy, conflict? Or is there something else?

Here we run again into the problem of the condensation of Freudian principles. Agency, fantasy, and conflict are central elements of Freud's original construction; as assumptions that organize clinical observation, they retain their clinical utility. Typically, however, they are not considered apart from an interpretive approach built on Freud's dual-instinct theory. The dual-instinct theory is a broad explanatory system that offers a particular way of understanding the observed phenomena, built on a set of assumptions about the child's motivations. It lays down a framework for ascribing a direction to the oedipal child's aims, a meaning to his fantasies, and a content to his conflicts. It answers a question that all analysts must ask: *What, ultimately, does the oedipal child want?*

The answer leads us further into our received version of the Oedipus complex. I have quite deliberately presented an account of the Oedipus complex without any mention at all of incest or parricide. Let me now suggest the relation of these themes to what I have discussed so far.

Relatively early in his career, Freud believed that he had found an explanation for the dramatic turn in the emotional lives of three- to six-year-olds. Each and every one of us is fated to relive, in our psychic reality, the destiny of the legendary Oedipus. Incest and parricide, the core of the Oedipus myth as Sophocles interpreted it, were actual occurrences in human prehistory. Now they are our phylogenetic heritage. Through evolutionary processes, generational conflict instigated by the incestuous and parricidal motives of the young has become a universal feature of mental life.

Freud, of course, provided an ontogeny of the Oedipus complex alongside his phylogenetic vision. In the individual child, oedipal motives emerge as a function of libidinal maturation. The child's phallic position lies behind the nature of his desire and of his experience generally. The impact of the phallic stage takes two forms. First, it determines the nature of the oedipal libidinal impulse: incestuous sexual intercourse. Second, the phallic aim is the first that supports or permits a whole-object relationship (1923a, p. 48). In this sense it contrasts with earlier developmental stages, which support only a relationship to a part-object such as the breast. Intercourse demands relatedness to the whole body of the other; thus the phallic child wants to possess *mother,* not just some part of her. For Freud

this development explains the more subtle interpersonal texture of the oedipal period. In the later history of psychoanalysis this advance in the quality of object relations was attributed partly to the maturation of the ego, but the centrality of libidinal determinants has never been superseded.

Although Freud's view of the role of aggression in the unfolding of the Oedipus complex never evolved as fully as his explanations in terms of libidinal development, the child's innate hostility is understood to cause his experience of rivalry. Oedipal fears are based, ultimately, on two factors: projection of aggressive impulses onto the (temporarily) hated parent, and assumptions that both competitively sexual and aggressive aims will be responded to punitively, according to the law of talion. For Freud, the phenomenology of the Oedipus complex is explicable as a vicissitude of libido and aggression.

Freud's drive theory addresses what the oedipal child wants and needs. It provided Freud with a motor for the Oedipus complex and guided his clinical understanding of the events through which it was enacted. According to the drive theory, the oedipal child is struggling—fundamentally and irreducibly—with sexual and murderous urges. Viewing the Oedipus complex this way relegates other human concerns—orality, narcissism, anal aggressiveness, merger fantasies, experiences of self-disintegration, and so on—to secondary or "preoedipal" status. These are then interpreted as defensive regressions from frightening incestuous and parricidal impulses.

In contemporary debate over the centrality of the Oedipus complex, incest and parricide dominate the discussion at the expense of the more interesting propositions concerning agency, fantasy, and conflict. Consider the way that Charles Brenner presents the Oedipus complex: "This, then, in briefest summary, is the full statement of what we call the oedipus complex. It is a twofold attitude toward both parents: on the one hand a wish to eliminate the jealously hated father and take his place in a sensual relationship with the mother, and on the other hand a wish to eliminate the jealously hated mother and take her place with the father" (1955, p. 118).

Nor is Brenner's statement atypical. In his comprehensive textbook of psychoanalytic theory, Fenichel was able to muster only these punning words by way of definition: "the Oedipus complex can be called the climax of infantile sexuality . . . erogenous development . . . culminate[s] in the Oedipus strivings, which as a rule are expressed by guilt-laden genital mas-

turbation. An overcoming of these strivings, to be replaced by adult sexuality, is the prerequisite for normality" (1945, p. 91).

Again, Robert Waelder has expressed a similarly one-sided interpretation: "All that the theory of the oedipus complex claims to be universally valid is the proposition that at the height of childhood sexuality—the phallic period—the boy's inborn phallic desires and his inborn or acquired aggressive or competitive strivings—are attached to the adults who rear the child, or to fantasied objects with which he may fill in the vacancies" (1960, p. 113). Moore and Fine, in their dictionary of psychoanalytic terms, elaborate the point: "During the phallic period the child strives for a sexual union (conceived variously according to the child's cognitive capacities) with the parent of the opposite sex and wishes for the death or disappearance of the parent of the same sex" (1990, p. 133).

This idea, that oedipal dynamics reflect the phase-specific workings of sexual and destructive impulses, has become the litmus test of theoretical orthodoxy; it is the new shibboleth. More important for the conceptual development of psychoanalysis, *a particular explanation of the Oedipus complex has become the Oedipus complex*. Analysts who organize their understanding of the ontogeny of human nature around events that are accessible to verbal memory, experiences that are significantly influenced by internally motivated fantasy, goals that have an organized direction but are inevitably conflicted, relationships that involve the child and both parents simultaneously—in short, analysts who wish to preserve the descriptive and functional centrality of oedipal dynamics—also adhere to the explanatory principles of the libido/aggression theory. Conversely, those who consider that phallic incestuous strivings and their more or less disguised expression in genital masturbation do not constitute an adequate foundation for building a theory of personality and its pathology reject the Oedipus complex in its entirety. Mitchell (1984, 1988) has aptly termed this theoretical strategy the "developmental tilt"—it avoids reductionist explanation at the expense of losing much that is valuable.

IT IS time for psychoanalysis to emerge from Freud's shadow. A century of clinical observation warrants construction of a new Oedipus complex— one built on our own experience, not simply out of a reflexive relation to the founder. A vignette will suggest the issues that this new formulation must address.

A boy in his early teens is playing tennis with his father. They have

played together—infrequently—for years, and the father has always won. Now there comes a day when the boy wins for the first time. The father reacts by announcing that he is getting old, never played very well in the first place, and might as well hang up his racket: he's through with tennis. He never plays again, either with his son or with friends.

The boy remembers the incident into adulthood and into his analysis. What is lost, however, is the depth of his emotions and, therefore, the significance of the whole story. That is, the boy loses, through repression, the sense of how his victory over his father activated impulses that we conceptualize in terms of ambition, self-assertion, joyous and collegial competitiveness, hostile and destructive competitiveness, sexual rivalry, and so on. At the same time, he will repress the attendant fears of losing his father, harming his father, surpassing his father. For the boy, the tennis match was a benchmark in becoming a man in a world of other men, but the whole thing is irretrievably distorted because winning was an act of murder as well as a sign of growth.

The incident gives rise not only to impulses and fears but also to images. The boy is apt to construct a representation of his father as fragile, vulnerable, and prone to retaliate with guilt-inducing, passive-aggressive self-destructiveness. As his associations to the particular situation reverberate through his experience, the boy will focus on a range of ideas about his family. He will recall images drawn from his relationship to his mother, from his impression of the mother's relationship to his father, even from what he has seen or inferred about his mother's relationship to her own father. Each evoked image contributes to the boy's feelings about his own capacity (not to say wish) to play with, to compete with, to destroy, and to replace his father. All the images, no less than the boy's wishes and fears, are likely to be repressed.

Consider the conflicts that are apparent even in this brief description of a typically "oedipal" event. The boy is attached to his father by needs of various kinds (that is, needs for all the gratifications and feelings of security that come from being a father's son) as well as by virtue of his love, loyalty, and concern. All of this assures that the father's continued well-being is important to the boy. At the same time, winning the match serves equally important aims: the boy is ambitious and wants to be competent, he is competitive and wants to win, he resents the years of subordination to his father and wants revenge, he harbors hostility and wants to defeat (even at times kill) his father. In addition to these conflicting motives the boy is buffeted by other irreconcilable images. He sees his father as strong,

angry, and vengeful and, at the same time, as weak, destructible, pushed over the edge by the simple fact of the boy's own growth.

Although the relationship between son and father moves to the foreground in the particular incident, the mother's role colors all that has happened. Her feelings about both men—who should be the stronger, who should be the survivor—provide a crucial backdrop for the event. If, for example, the mother is committed (wishfully and/or by virtue of judgment) to a vision of her husband as weak and her son as heir to male potency within her own family, conflicts both of loyalty and of self-interest will plague the boy. Winning attaches him to his mother and her hopes, even as it separates him from and betrays his father. Or perhaps winning is a submission—in the act of triumph, the boy feels that he loses his autonomy by serving his mother's purpose. The very meaning of competence and individuation will be conflicted in the boy's experience.

Although I have drawn this vignette from a transaction characterized predominantly by the father's dramatic reaction to losing, it should be clear that the boy's feelings and conflicts, although intensified by the event, were not caused by it. Winning for the first time is not and cannot be an unambivalent experience. Just as even the proudest father senses his own decline in the loss, the son inevitably feels twinges of sympathy, guilt, and remorse. Also he will sense the anxiety that comes from knowing that he has defeated a strong protector, and that the next step takes him farther away from the safety and comforts of home.

Even in the best of circumstances, it is unlikely that these feelings will be identified as such by either participant, although they will briefly enter awareness and be the stuff of the ineffable sadness that intrudes on every celebration. But the vignette highlights those experiences—inevitably fantastically elaborated and interpersonally enacted—that characterize the crucial growth experience called the Oedipus complex.

On the assumption that the tennis match condenses a series of experiences that are central to this boy's development, later in life he is likely to become inhibited in pursuing motives seen as the prerogative of adult males. His analysis would certainly be devoted to work on "oedipal" themes. But it would be misleading to assume—as those who confuse the Oedipus complex with the drive-theory explanation of it would—that the conflicts originate exclusively or even predominantly in the boy's sexual and aggressive fantasies and his defenses against them. This narrow approach simply cannot stand up to what we know clinically.

Even more important, treating this boy-become-patient principally with

a view to uncovering his incestuous and parricidal goals would seriously miscarry the analytic process. In fact, it would be fair to say that the presenting problem—the inhibition—stems from a *fear* that self-assertion or ambition or competitiveness or masculinity itself are inevitably incestuous and murderous. Interpretations rooted in drive theory, by confirming these fears, can strengthen a harsh superego and thus reduce anxiety, often with considerable symptomatic improvement. They do not, on that account, constitute a complete analysis.

A new Oedipus complex would recognize the range and complexity of motives, emotions, and impressions that contribute to the formation of this central developmental event. But, as it gets away from the restrictive and misleading confines of the libido/aggression theory, the new Oedipus complex avoids the excesses of Freud's more strident critics. Heinz Kohut, as perhaps the most well-known critic in recent years, emphasized the interplay of ambition and admiration in the oedipal drama, both of which clearly play a part in my vignette. But Kohut's anti-Freudian zeal led him away from the wisdom of the original construct. Thus he saw exuberance as the "normal" emotion of the oedipal years, viewing any departure as evidence of psychopathology, caused by parental failure to react appropriately to the developing child's new capacities. Kohut lost sight of the conflicts caused by the advent of these capacities or by the changes in intimate relationships that must accompany growth. Further, he could not include any sense of the oedipal child as an agent of his conflictual experiences. The child's motives are unitary; any thwarting must come from outside.

Clinicians know that wishes to exercise newly acquired capacities, like incestuous and parricidal impulses, are motivational components of the Oedipus complex. And exuberance, guilt, shame, and mourning are characteristic emotions of the oedipal years. Growth, becoming a person among other people, is inevitably conflictual; every gain entails some loss. But in conceptualizing these conflicts, existing theory lags sadly behind clinical wisdom. The institutionalization of theoretical constructs bequeaths us an unhappy choice between narrowness and naiveté.

Drive Concepts

The Interpretive System of Psychoanalysis

THE OEDIPUS complex is the greatest monument we have to the timeless power of childhood. Etched forever in the unconscious, oedipal wishes, fears, fantasies, and impressions continue to shape experience throughout life. Clinically, the Oedipus complex remains the most effective tool for talking to adult patients about their archaic past. It provides a powerful link between contemporary psychopathology and its prehistoric roots.

But, as I have argued, the clinical experience of many analysts has raised questions about whether it is possible to think of oedipal phenomena simply as derivatives of the child's incestuous and parricidal wishes. Thus the continuing influence of one of Freud's great inventions, the Oedipus complex, is threatened by the persistence of another of his great inventions, the libido/aggression theory. It is time for psychoanalysts to acknowledge this tension and to unravel the difficulties in the relation between the Oedipus complex and the dual-instinct theory. To do this, we must reexamine the role of drive in the conceptual system of psychoanalysis.

A comment of Freud's will help us to begin. In a passage from *New Introductory Lectures on Psycho-Analysis,* he succinctly summarizes the development of psychoanalysis from its clinical origins to the elaboration of its theoretical structure. "The path," he writes, "led from symptoms to the unconscious, to the life of the instincts, to sexuality" (1933, p. 57). My goal in this chapter will be to suggest the implications of Freud's division of that path into three individual steps. Understanding how he moved from his clinical observations to the drive model will illuminate the relation between his abstract metapsychological formulations and the in-

terpretive implications of classical psychoanalysis. It will also highlight the
strengths and weaknesses of Freud's vision.

The path Freud followed led him to create a distinctive interpretive
system. His drive theory became what Schafer (1983) has called a "storyline," a narrative structure that defines the data of observation and shapes
them into a psychoanalytic construction. I believe that looking at the drive
theory in this way will prove useful, although it is rather unconventional.
Usually when analysts think about the drives, what they have in mind is
something organismic. Drives are seen as a quasi-physiological force, stirrings within us handed down from our bestial beginnings and associated
with what is most inchoate in our behavior. Because they are our evolutionary heritage, the drives bridge a border between psychology and biology. Freud occasionally, and especially Hartmann after him, argued for the
validity of the drive model on biological rather than clinical grounds. Apparently the drives are the stuff of phylogeny, not of narrative.

But despite its presumed roots in biology—actually a controversial issue
in its own right and one to which I will return in Chapter 4—the drives
can be studied as psychological forces. Accordingly, theorists have also
understood the narrative power of drive. Rudolph Loewenstein said that
drive reveals the *direction* of mental life (1940). Edward Bibring was more
explicit. Once Freud evolved his final dual-instinct theory with its broad
focus on the tendencies toward life and death:

> instinct was not a tension of energy which impinged upon the mental sphere,
> which arose from an organic source and which aimed at removing a state of
> excitation in the organ from which it originated. It was a directive or directed
> "something" which guided the life processes in a certain direction (Bibring,
> 1936, p. 128).

Giving the same view a clinical slant, Hartmann noted that, because it is
the force underlying all behavior, drive is the source of psychological pattern. Without some concept like drive, psychoanalytic investigation itself
would be impossible (1948). With this approach in mind, I will follow
Freud along the steps on his path.

Step 1: From symptoms to the unconscious. The first step—today, of course,
we would refer not only to symptoms but to all those characteristics that
define the individual personality—is accepted by all analysts. The very
concept of a therapeutically beneficial psychoanalytic inquiry, which as-

sumes that one can effect change by broadening patients' awareness of their experience, would make no sense without an underlying conviction that aspects of experience are kept from consciousness in ordinary circumstances.

This became apparent as soon as anybody tried to do clinical psychoanalytic work. From the beginning, thinking about patients psychoanalytically meant assuming that their symptoms were motivated. But—confoundingly—the patients could not name their motives, any more than subjects of hypnotic experiments could name the reasons for their strange post-hypnotic behaviors. Exposed by analytic inquiry, the motives themselves turned out to be quite ordinary; they were the hopes, fears, and feelings of everyday life. What made them extraordinary was precisely that the patients could not easily become aware of them. There was a nearly impenetrable barrier between these unconscious ideas and other mental contents.

In Freud's original formulations, this barrier defined the border of the dynamic unconscious (or "the repressed"). The unconscious began as a structural (or, as he called it then, topographic) concept—it referred to a region of the mind. It is helpful to think of the early unconscious as a kind of container; Freud himself compared it to a large room (1916–17, p. 245). The container can be filled with any mental content that for some reason patients could not accept as fully their own. Freud began psychoanalytic theorizing by creating a container. Only later did he insist that the container was filled with specific contents. The work of filling the container was left to later stages.

Step 2: From the dynamic unconscious to instinct, or drive. The concept of drive broadly stated—stated, that is, in the terms of Loewenstein, Bibring, and Hartmann—implies the following: There are conceptually irreducible, endogenous forces at work within us that operate as prime movers of the mind and that decisively shape all human experience. All mental activity begins with the stirring of some internal need. This is what drive is conceptually—an unconditioned internal need that motivates all behavior and determines the quality of all experience. Note that to this point the formulation of drive implies neither an a priori nor an empirical judgment about what these instinctual needs might be or about what the person might do to satisfy them. That is what Freud meant by distinguishing this step on his path from step 3, "from instincts to sexuality." Step 2 does, however, have crucial interpretive implications of its own.

An example suggested in a slightly different context by Roy Schafer (1985) will illuminate these implications. Schafer describes a patient who, in the course of his associations, says, "My father is old." This comment conveys information to the analyst—but what is the information about? The intuitive answer is that the patient is simply telling us something that is true about his father. That sort of literal listening, however, does not take the unconscious into account.

If we are listening to the patient with unconscious influences in mind, we will consider that the referents of the comment go beyond the specifics of what has been said. On the one hand, we may think that age is a metaphor, that the patient is using it as a way of expressing his less palatable concerns about his father's weakness, apathy, passivity, depression, or victimization within the family. Similarly, the reference to the father as the object of the patient's experience may itself be metaphorical. The patient may be making a disguised reference to somebody else—the analyst himself comes to mind.

Although no analyst would take the patient's comment purely at face value, there are significant differences when it comes to conceptualizing the source of the impression. For some analysts the impression is, inevitably, based in the patient's interpersonal experience. It may originate in something he has recognized about his father or about somebody else; and it may be organized around the other person's age or around something else. But it is anchored in observations of others and says something about what these observations are.

Freud was never satisfied with this way of understanding his patients' thoughts. He insisted on taking an additional step, on asking a further question about the patient's need to experience things in a particular way and to report the experience to the analyst at a particular time. Asking this question led Freud away from interpersonal perception. The patient's thought that his father was old could not be explained by the fact that he *was* old (or by anything else about the father). After all, our impressions of others are always highly subjective. Freud insisted that the experience of *father* is driven from inside. The patient's association can only convey information about the patient, about current needs, fears, and conflicts.

Constructing either/or choices is always disconcerting. Can't we have it both ways, at least clinically? Isn't any good analyst going to be concerned *both* with the impression *and* with the need? I think not. For one thing, the way the analyst hears the patient's association will determine the next

question that comes to mind. An analyst working with Freud's sensibility would wonder next, internally or out loud: "Why would the patient, just now, be thinking of his father (or, by displacement, about someone else, such as the analyst) this way?" An analyst who did not accept the internal origin of all experience would go in quite a different direction. She might ask: "What is it like for this patient, being the child of an old father (or the patient of an old analyst)?" Each question sets the analytic inquiry on its own particular course.

These alternative questions are the clinical tip of a philosophical iceberg. They reflect the issues involved in an age-old dispute about the nature of human experience. The terms of this issue within philosophy were clearly set out in the debate between the British empiricists (most prominently Hume and Locke) and the continental rationalists (Descartes and Leibniz).

The empiricists held that there is no possibility of knowledge independent of what we learn through our perception of the external world, and that our perceptions themselves are unconditionally imprinted on the mind as one writes on a blank slate. In 1734 Hume questioned how we can know that one event causes another. We can observe that, when one billiard ball hits another, the second moves. But can we say with any legitimate conviction that the impact caused the movement? We can see the two events, and we can remember that in our own experience one event invariably follows the other. But where in this is a *cause*? The cause is an inference, a product of reason, and reason can always be faulty. We can only be sure of what we learn through our senses. Inner mental processes are always suspect.

The rationalists turned this argument on its head. Sensory information can never be trusted, they said. After all, many perceptions turn out to be illusory—we learn that lesson every day when we wake up from a dream. All we can count on for sure is our awareness of what goes on inside our heads. When Descartes insists "I think, therefore I am," he is beginning with the bedrock certainty of his own cognition. The next step, that there must be a thing in the world "out there" that does the thinking, is a deduction. The world of sensory data can never be known directly—it can only be inferred.

The contrast is clear, and it is dichotomous. The empiricists assert that only the external world can be known, that we must forever be skeptical about the world of the mind. The rationalists insist that only our inner

experience is trustworthy, that perception is unavoidably suspect. The dichotomy itself is inherent in attempts to grapple with the nature of human experience.*

The debate continues in contemporary psychoanalysis. The empiricist position is reflected in the sensibility of relational theorists. Consider two comments of Edgar Levenson, who advocates an extreme empiricism. Mocking many analysts' claims to infer their patients' hidden inner motives and fantasies, Levenson suggests: "'Dynamics,' as psychoanalysts use it, is the attribution of purpose to behavior, and behavior is defined by the therapist's hermeneutics—by what he thinks matters" (1972, p. 207). Attempts to penetrate the inner world of the mind are little more than an analytic conceit; we would be better off to stick with what can be surely known. Thus, "For the Freudian, the key question is, what does it truly mean? For the interpersonalist, the question is, what's going on around here?" (1985, p. 53).

But, as always, skepticism is a two-way street. Contemporary drive theorists uphold the rationalist tradition. Inner processes can be known, they argue. That is the fundamental premise of psychoanalytic inquiry. Problems arise when we claim certainty about the external world. Thus Jacob Arlow writes: "We can apply reality testing to the physical attributes of people, but once we begin to apply the concept of reality to interpersonal relations and to the total social milieu, we introduce variables that are not easily tested, that elude simple, confirmable definition" (1985a, p. 524). Psychoanalytic theorists today are struggling with the same epistemological dichotomy that has plagued philosophers for centuries.

For Freud, psychoanalytic investigation was a practical application of rationalist epistemological sensibilities. Ultimately, he insisted, experience must be traced to its innermost origins—to what he considered the "depths" of the mind. Consider how he reacted to his patient Dora when she criticized her father. Although he could agree that much of what Dora had to say was correct, Freud could not let himself stop with acknowledging the interpersonal reality. He insisted: "A string of reproaches against other people leads one to suspect the existence of a string of self-

---

*There is a middle road in the philosophical debate. It was proposed in 1781 by Immanuel Kant, who taught that although all knowledge begins with perception, the perceptions themselves are conditioned by certain characteristics of the human mind. David Rapaport (1947, 1959) and Samuel Novey (1957) have argued for the affinity of Freudian and Kantian sensibilities. But I believe that in the final analysis Freud tilts away from a balanced Kantian approach to a more committed and doctrinaire rationalism.

reproaches with the same content" (1905b, p. 35). The patient's perception of others, *however accurate,* is essentially an externalization, what
Freud later in the same passage described as an "automatic . . . method of
defending oneself."

Certainly Freud was as relentless with himself as he was with his patients. In interpreting his own dreams, he invariably worked inward. The
manifest content of the dreams, or at least his first associations to them,
often related to his perceptions of others. But Freud's interpretive path
immediately led him away from this aspect of his experience, which he
consistently dismissed as superficial. Having skirted his observations,
Freud arrived quickly at what he considered an attempt to justify his own
behavior, and finally at a self-criticism for something he had done or
wished to do.

Although it has powerful interpretive possibilities, sometimes Freud's
preference led him to stunningly partial explanations of his dreams. Consider the now famous dream he had around the time of his father's funeral.
The dream consists only of the image of a placard bearing a message about
which Freud is uncertain. It says either "You are requested to close the
eyes" or "You are requested to close an eye." Freud's first association is
that the phrase refers to "overlook[ing]" or "wink[ing] at" something
(1900, p. 318).

It seems inescapable that there is some reference in this to not speaking,
or thinking, ill of the dead. Like the patient who says "My father is old,"
Freud's dream appears to convey some information about his father—
information that Freud finds difficult to confront directly. In fact, there is
a great deal of evidence suggesting that the problem of knowing all there
was to know about his father is one with which Freud struggled mightily
(Gay, 1988; Krüll, 1986). Recall that he abandoned his seduction
theory—on which he had staked his career—when he realized that if it
were true it must mean that "in every case the father, not excluding my
own, had to be blamed as a pervert" (1950, letter 69, p. 259). Evidently
even this sacrifice was not quite enough. Six weeks after renouncing the
theory in a letter to his friend Wilhelm Fliess, he has returned to the problem and further disposed of it. He writes again to Fliess describing a state
of inner excitement and discovery:

> I can only say . . . that *der Alte* [my father] played no active part in my case,
> but that no doubt I drew an inference by analogy from myself on to him;
> that the "prime originator" [of my troubles] was a woman, ugly, elderly, but
> clever (1950, letter 70, p. 261).

Freud's father is off the hook with this revelation, and the blame for Freud's neurosis is shared by his ugly old nurse and (later on in the story) by the premature stirrings of his own libido.

The exoneration of Freud *père* runs throughout the dream analysis. Freud never even considers the possibility that he is telling himself in the dream to wink at something he knows or could know about his father. Instead he quickly concludes that he is reproaching himself for overlooking his own behavior. He finds two reasons to blame himself: he had arranged a simple funeral, and he arrived slightly late at the house of mourning (1950, letter 50, p. 233). These seem like petty failings at a time when the emotional stakes are high; it is unlikely that they can fully explain such a striking dream. This is especially true in light of the facts Freud reports. His lateness was caused by external circumstances and, most impressively, the simple funeral reflected his father's own stated preference (1900, p. 318). Nevertheless, Freud concludes that "the dream is an outlet for the inclination to self-reproach which is regularly present among the survivors" (1950, p. 233).*

Freud's interpretive preference is reflected theoretically in his embrace of the rationalist sensibility. Generalizing his clinical interest in getting beyond the reproach to the self-reproach, he was continually at pains to remind us that perceptions of what goes on around us are never so important as those arising from within. Internal perceptions, he claims, "are more primordial, more elementary, than perceptions arising externally . . . [they have] greater economic significance" (1923a, p. 22).

This is the background for Freud's definition of instinct as a "demand made upon the mind for work" and for his dictum that it is "the ultimate cause of all activity." Having defined the unconscious with step 1, in step 2 he has gone on to take a strong position about the origin and nature of all experience. This stand has important implications for our expectations about what we will find when we probe the unconscious psychoanalytically. What we will find—if we use Freud's method correctly—comes down finally to transformations of the basic needs that characterize human nature. We will find specific impulses and more fully articulated motives that seek to satisfy these needs; we will find memories that are organized

---

*Probably the most famous example of the interpretive style I am describing can be found in the most famous dream in psychoanalysis. Interpreting the dream of Irma's injection (1900), Freud unearths a self-reproach in place of what clearly could be a fatal indictment of his friend Fliess. The story of the dramatic events leading up to this dream is told well by Peter Gay (1988).

around their frustration or gratification; we will find images (self and object representations) that embody the history of attempts to achieve instinctual satisfaction.

But always, when the analysis is complete, we will find the undisguised, untransformed need itself. Fenichel put it this way: "noninstinctual mental phenomena are derivatives of more primitive instinctual ones" (1945, p. 12). It is the rationalist view of mind, given a psychological meaning and requiring a specific clinical commitment. But as Freud makes clear, insisting on a rationalist position does not imply any particular judgment about what the drives themselves are. That judgment requires a further step, one he did not take until he had been working clinically for more than a decade.

Step 3: From the life of the instincts to sexuality. Having insisted on the existence of some endogenous prime mover of the mind, Freud was left with the problem of specifying the qualities and aims of the fundamental drives. Each of the many possibilities carried its own strengths and weaknesses. Freud could be modest about his choices. In "Instincts and Their Vicissitudes" he wrote:

> What instincts should we suppose there are, and how many? . . . I have proposed that two groups of . . . primal instincts should be distinguished . . . But this supposition has not the status of a necessary postulate . . . it is merely a working hypothesis, to be retained only so long as it proves useful (1915a, pp. 123–124).

In his second dual-instinct theory Freud chose sexuality and aggression as his motivational and experiential first principles. This is the most controversial step along the path. One can follow Freud even as far as instinct without following him to the primacy of sexuality and aggression. Many analysts have suggested alternative theories: dependency drives, competence or mastery drives, drives for self-cohesion, and drives for individuation are prominent in the literature, along with many others. Generally, however, the theorists who proposed these alternatives have been relegated to the role of dissenter.

Freud's theoretical decision to place sexuality at the core of his motivational system was rooted in some early therapeutic successes. The history of these successes is worth reviewing briefly, by way of reminding ourselves how he got to step 3 on his path. Psychoanalytic theorizing began, early in the course of the investigation of hysterical symptoms, with Joseph Breuer's discovery of the therapeutic value of patients telling their

thoughts to a therapist. These investigations took as their data mental contents and meanings. It turned out that the pathology of hysteria consisted of meanings which, by virtue of subjectively irreconcilable conflicts with other meanings, had been banished from consciousness. As might be expected, improvement came about when meanings were redefined and reshuffled, thereby undoing the pathogenic mix. This was termed the "talking cure" and was conceived of technically as making the unconscious conscious. From the patients' perspective, what happened was that the ability to be aware of their own mental contents greatly increased, broadening the perspective on the meaning of their experience.

In his earliest formulations Freud makes it clear that virtually any two meanings may conflict with each other, provoking the trauma that is at the root of neurosis (1894, 1896b); the step on Freud's path from the unconscious to instinct was yet to be taken. If there was any notion of a drive at all, it was implicit, and it was represented—oddly enough—by what Freud then called the ego. The ego of 1895 embodies the only constant motivational force in human experience. A composite of conscious ideas, the ego worked like a drive because it guided experience and behavior in a consistent direction.

The ego of 1895 prefigures the instinct of self-preservation. The "dominant mass of ideas" includes those ideas that express the person's adaptive needs—both the need for safety in a literal, physical sense (Breuer and Freud, 1895, p. 9) and the need for what Rapaport calls "social propriety and self-respect" (1959, p. 18). Any experience that threatened the ongoing feeling of well-being would, if certain other conditions were met, be likely to undergo repression and thus exert a pathogenic effect.

As he gathered experience with the psychoanalytic method, Freud became progressively more convinced that the meanings that threatened the sense of well-being, and therefore the meanings that were likely to become embroiled in conflict with adaptive trends, were exclusively sexual. Therapeutic success depended on uncovering the repressed sexual experience. Freud's insistence on probing deeper—at the time "deeper" meant further into the archaic past—eventually led him to construct the seduction theory (1896a, 1896b, 1896c, 1898). Once the seduction theory was in place, Freud had a working model of the conflicts that were central to the transference neuroses (though this was far more modest than the generalized conflict theory he came to years later). Neurotic conflict always consisted of some sexual meaning (a wish, an impulse, a memory), on one side, and the need for adaptive social living on the other.

Even as he was working on unraveling the mysteries of hysterical symptoms, Freud was engaged in another undertaking: the creation of a "scientific" psychology on a par with other natural sciences. His work in this area was based on the conventional view of mind at the time: it was a passive structure energized by external stimuli. Because he viewed the mind as an energized structure, Freud needed an energy source. He made two early attempts to locate it, neither of which quite satisfied him. First he equated energy with affect, and affect was simply the individual's emotional reaction to events. Next, with the first published theory of the general workings of the mind in chapter 7 of *The Interpretation of Dreams,* he suggested that the mind is energized by wishes. Wishes are instigated by disturbances of homeostasis that are caused by surges of tension stemming from need. The wish is a desire to recreate the circumstances in which similar needs have been satisfactorily met in the past. Freud does not say much about the nature of the wishes or about what the underlying needs are. He refers only to "the exigencies of life," implying that they could be almost anything (1900, p. 565).

The theoretical problem of an energy source converged with the clinical problems of psychoanalysis when Freud publicly abandoned his early views on the role of sexuality in the etiology of the neuroses (1905a and especially 1906). The seduction theory could no longer be sustained, he declared. He had to acknowledge that his patients' reports of childhood seductions were not necessarily true. This failure of theoretical expectation challenged what had until then apparently been a comfortably empiricist position on the origin of experience. Seduction was a real event in the external world; it was *"an actual irritation of the genitals"* occurring before puberty (1896b, p. 163, original italics). Unconscious contents—particularly the memories recovered in the course of analysis—were assumed to be the representations of actual events.

I refer to Freud's early empiricist sensibilities as "apparent." For some time he had serious doubts. In the letter to Fliess announcing the failure of his seduction theory (fully eight years before he announced it publicly), Freud wrote of "the certain discovery that there are no indications of reality in the unconscious, so that one cannot distinguish between the truth and fiction that is cathected with affect" (1950, letter 69, p. 260). These early doubts coalesced by 1905 into the concept of a psychic reality. The key element in the construction of the idea of psychic reality was the theory of instinctual drive, particularly the theory of the sexual drive. What patients repressed were not memories of actual events—they were

fantasies that were the derivatives in experience of innate, maturationally unfolding drives. The energy of these drives, the force behind the impulse, in turn provided the fuel for the operation of the mind.

In *Three Essays on the Theory of Sexuality* Freud argued that psychic energy moves the mind (and the person) in a particular direction. Put another way, the instinctual impulse has a specific *content*, precisely the content he had found in conflicts that lay behind the transference neuroses. On one side of the conflict, the transposition of sexual events from outer reality (the seductions) to inner reality (the impulses that arose endogenously along with their ramifications) is quite literal. And on the other side were the requirements to live safely and adaptively, demands represented by the dominant mass of ideas. Both facets of the conflict were enshrined metapsychologically as instincts. Freud summarized it years later by saying that the "facts could be met by drawing a contrast between the sexual instincts and ego instincts *(instincts of self-preservation)*, which was in line with the popular saying that hunger and love are what make the world go round" (1923b, p. 255).

With this, Freud took the final step on the path he outlined. Sexuality (always the more interesting drive to Freud) was firmly in place as the primary, irreducible, endogenous force underlying not only all motivated behavior but also the construction of psychic reality. Libido was, as Thomas Ogden has usefully described it, "the Rosetta stone which allows the human being to translate raw sensory data into meaning-laden experience" (1984, p. 507). It was the keystone of Freud's rationalist vision of mind. In the 1920 revision of the dual-instinct theory, and especially in the elaboration of the revision by Hartmann, Kris, and Loewenstein, aggression was given an equal or nearly equal role in the psychic economy. This evolution gave us the fundamental conceptual structure that remains the basis of Freudian drive theory.

What Drive Is Not

Joseph Smith had his tongue only slightly in cheek when he wrote, "Unconscious instinctual drives as the ultimate motives of behavior was the idea that changed the world" (1986, p. 546). Certainly there is a compelling grandeur to Freud's vision of man driven, and driven mad, by passions that he is fated to master at best only incompletely. Robert Waelder wrote of the "imperative, majestic, power of *Trieb*," and not only the drive impulse but the theory itself stirs fervent excitement (1960, p. 98).

Because it is so imposing, there is a tendency, among some analysts as

well as among interested lay people, to confuse the libido/aggression theory with the whole of Freudian psychoanalysis. Many analysts overlook Freud's description of his theoretical path as involving three distinct steps. In this section I will take up two common misconceptions that result from merging theoretical propositions that ought to be kept independent. These are, first, that rejecting the libido/aggression theory means rejecting the existence of a dynamic unconscious (a mistake that results from collapsing steps 1 and 2 on Freud's path); and second, that rejecting the libido/aggression theory means minimizing the importance of sexual and aggressive motives in the conduct of human life (a mistake resulting from collapsing steps 2 and 3).

Any theorist who rejects drive theory has rejected the dynamic unconscious. Commenting on Freud's personal attitudes toward his creation, Smith says that Freud "preferred to think that what all the fuss was about was simply that, by a stroke of genius and luck, he had hit upon a new field, one that dethroned consciousness and brought sexuality to the fore" (1986, p. 545). In Smith's view, it took only one stroke to establish both the unconscious and a drive theory.

Smith doesn't do so, but it is easy to use this formulation polemically. Once accepted, it becomes a weapon for excluding dissidents from psychoanalytic dialogue on the ground that they have discarded the system's most essential hypothesis. Consider a paper by Homer Curtis. In a summary statement about heterodox theorists ranging from Horney to Sullivan to Fromm to Kohut to Balint, he concludes that "with the exception of the schools of Jung and Melanie Klein the predominant trend in the various alternate theories is away from the centrality of the dynamic unconscious and toward the environment and interpersonal elements in the neurotic equation" (1985, p. 340).

What Curtis has done is to substitute a definition of the unconscious in terms of its contents for a more structurally based definition that stays true to the steps on the path Freud described. He evidently believes that speaking of the dynamic unconscious is equivalent to speaking about aspects of experience that arise internally. Thus he has confused the concept of an unconscious with a rationalist view of mind. Although he is uncommonly tendentious about it, Curtis' misunderstanding is not particularly unusual. In their dictionary of psychoanalytic terms, LaPlanche and Pontalis argue that the notion of specific contents is one of the "essential characteristics of the unconscious as a system" (1973, p. 474).

There is some truth to this, but it is limited. Charles Brenner is certainly

correct when he writes that, as Freud's clinical experience developed, he realized that unconscious contents were more diverse than he had expected them to be (1955, p. 37). When he first defined the unconscious (systemic Ucs.) in chapter 7 of *The Interpretation of Dreams* Freud did say that its contents were limited to infantile wishes and their repressed derivatives. But this represents only a moment in the evolution of psychoanalytic theory; there was an unconscious before chapter 7, and there was an unconscious later on. Earlier, in the *Studies on Hysteria,* unconscious contents included impulses, memories, fears, attitudes, wishes, plans—anything incompatible with the dominant mass of ideas. Then there was a phase during which only wishes could be unconscious, and another during which the wishes themselves had to be based in sexual impulses. Later Freud acknowledged the existence of unconscious defenses and of the unconscious affects that triggered them (mainly anxiety and guilt). By the time of the *New Introductory Lectures* Freud was even referring to "impressions . . . which have been sunk into the id by repression" (1933, p. 74). These changes highlight the value of thinking of the unconscious as a container—one that Freud filled with whatever contents he found as his clinical experience grew. The unconscious itself cannot be defined by or equated with any notion about contents.

Consider the problems that arise from Curtis' misunderstanding. He is unable to distinguish alternative psychoanalytic models from psychological theories that genuinely reject the concept of unconscious experience and thus preclude the kind of inquiry that defines psychoanalytic treatment. Thus he misunderstands the fundamental contributions of theorists who have argued against the rationalist (drive-theoretical) position within psychoanalysis. Of those theorists he mentions, all but Sullivan centrally argue for unconscious as well as conscious determinants of behavior and for a repression barrier that sets up a dynamic tension between the two. Even Sullivan, whose stylistic preference guided him away from such reifiable concepts as *the* unconscious, had conceptual ideas covering the same ground.

Jung and Klein, in whose work Curtis is able to find an unconscious, in fact share Freud's rationalist view of mind. Some dissident theorists, however, genuinely differ from Freud with respect to his rationalist perspective and its corresponding vision of unconscious contents. Many analysts believe that there are highly organized unconscious ideas—self and object representations, beliefs about relationships, and so on. These are based in the realities of interpersonal observation; they give rise to rather than

being derived from the unconscious wishes and impulses themselves. In significant respects, this approach characterizes theorizing within the relational model of the mind. One can see it clearly in Fairbairn's concept of internal objects, in Kohut's repressed self and object representations, and also in Sullivan's "personifications."

Among those who continue to declare at least some allegiance to the drive model, Otto Kernberg is a prominent exponent of the hypothesis that the unconscious can contain perceptions. This appears in his view that the repressed portion of the id consists of warded-off representations of the self in interaction with others (1976). Roy Schafer (1985) has written persuasively on the importance of unconscious communication and unconscious reality testing, and Theodore Dorpat (1985) has argued that much unconscious content derives from the denial of painful aspects of our interpersonal world. Joseph Sandler's recent proposal for a revised topographic model of the mind posits an unconscious containing complex representations of the self and its objects (Sandler and Sandler, 1987).

These hypotheses about unconscious contents represent genuinely psychoanalytic alternatives to Freud's rationalist vision; they are constructions based on data emerging from psychoanalytic inquiry. Saying that they are "environmental" and therefore not unconscious (as Curtis does) is a disservice to Freud and does great harm to the vitality of psychoanalysis as a discipline. It precludes the possibility of analysts ever learning anything new from their clinical experience.

Any theorist who rejects the libido/aggression theory underestimates the importance of sexuality and aggression as motives. It is hard to imagine that anyone could work clinically for any length of time without noticing how frequently people seek (often unconsciously) to gratify sexual or aggressive impulses. This observation would be predicted by the libido/aggression theory, but it would be a meager theory indeed if that was all it said. In truth it says far more. First, the libido/aggression theory asserts that *all* motives are ultimately reducible to sexual and aggressive impulses. Second, it claims that the sexual and aggressive impulses themselves are irreducible. The drive impulse is the primitive psychic unit. Its occurrence cannot be explained by any other psychological event.

Some analysts, attempting to preserve a political loyalty to the drive model while severing their conceptual ties to it, overlook these two fundamental meanings of the libido/aggression theory. Consider a comment of Sandler's:

the need for psychoanalysts to defend the significance of sexual and aggressive wishes has led to the building of theories in which everything tends to
be brought back to the drives. I am convinced that for most psychoanalysts
such reductionism plays a less significant part in their analytic work than in
their theory. What they are often much more concerned with are the variety
of *motives* for the use of defences, for the construction and development of
fantasies and transference . . . Certainly sexual and aggressive drives provide
highly important motives, but so do threats to our feelings of safety . . .
injuries to our self-esteem, feelings of guilt and shame, and threats from the
real ("external") world (1983, p. 42).

In this formulation, Sandler defines drive as one among many motives.
Drive refers simply to those motives that generate sexual and aggressive
activity. I agree strongly with Sandler's clinical idea that Freud's motivational system must be broadened. But this sensibility gets in the way of
his theoretical understanding. Sandler believes that bringing things "back
to the drives" reflects a defensive need of the analyst's. It does not; rather,
it is a central requirement of the drive concept itself. Drive theory asserts
that all motivated behavior must be explained, in the final analysis, as a
derivative or vicissitude of the drives. What else could Freud mean when
he describes the drives as "the ultimate cause of *all* activity"? What else
can Fenichel mean when he insists that *everything* is derived from instinct?

Fred Pine has also reconstrued the model, proposing a "drive psychology" as one of four independent motivational systems. The drive psychology is organized around "regularly recurring moments of need tension"
(1985, p. 63). These needs underlie some but not all of the child's (and
later the adult's) experience. Like Sandler, Pine argues that there is an
aspect of human functioning in which needs for the expression of sexual
and aggressive impulses dominate. But Pine's drive psychology is not the
libido/aggression theory. That theory does not simply maintain that some
behavior is directed toward sexual or aggressive goals—all of it is. Like
Sandler, Pine's clinical goals are admirable, but his approach muddies the
theoretical waters.

My objection to authors who believe that rejecting the libido/aggression
theory means rejecting the importance of sexuality and anger is more than
merely semantic. Both Sandler and Pine address one of the interpretive
constrictions of the model—its reductionism—so on this side of things
my criticism is mainly terminological. But there is a second, equally serious problem that neither addresses: the assumption that sexual and aggressive motives themselves are psychologically irreducible. If we reject

this assumption, if libido and aggression are not drives *in Freud's original sense,* then the interpreting analyst must look beyond the sexual or angry behaviors to find an explanation for their occurrence.

This, of course, is a fundamental requirement for relational theorists. Fairbairn and Kohut, each in his own way, explain impulsive, impersonal sexual and aggressive behaviors as the consequence of thwarted efforts to make contact with others. Mitchell (1988) offers a more evolved and elegant formulation of the relational motives underlying normal as well as perverse sexual expression. For Mitchell, sexuality expresses a wide range of personal and interpersonal themes. Therefore he finds fulfilled and not just thwarted relatedness at the core of sexual activity. Having rejected the premises of libido/aggression theory, Fairbairn, Kohut, and Mitchell are doing what they must do, conceptually and clinically. By retaining the term "drive" but not its definition or its meaning, Sandler and Pine are begging the most crucial psychoanalytic question.

What Drive Is

Because drive theory has become a political rallying cry as well as a clinical and theoretical tool, it can be hard to locate its actual contribution to the conceptual structure of psychoanalysis. It will help to clarify this contribution if we first look at four characteristics that define Freud's concept of drive.

1. Drive is a demand made on the mind for work. It is the only source of the energy that fuels the workings of mind. Put slightly differently, it is a way of conceptualizing our primary motivations. No matter how remote from instinctual aims it may seem to be, all behavior is ultimately derived from them.

2. Drive has a qualitatively specific nature manifested by its aims; they drive us in a particular direction. A crucial element of Freud's theory is that it is determinedly dualistic. There were always two drives in the system: first, sexual and self-preservative; later, the life and death instincts and their clinical manifestations, sexuality and aggression. Together, the two postulated drives exhaust man's pre-experiential motivational endowment; if they do not, there will be a motivational "hole" in the system, an indeterminacy that undermines the theory's explanatory power.

3. Drive aims precede experience; the drives are with us at birth and their nature is fixed phylogenetically. The distinction between the two drives (sexuality and self-preservations, or libido and aggression) is itself

pre-experiential. The drives as defined must be psychologically irreducible—they must not be capable of dissection into simpler elements on the basis of analytic evidence.

4. Drive is a constitutional variable. Drive endowment, the strength and balance of the two drives, differs among different individuals (see Freud, 1923a).

EARLIER I argued that the conceptual value of the Oedipus complex lies in its clinical implications. Specifically, the Oedipus complex embodies a view of human nature and its pathology based on the ubiquity of intrapsychic conflict, the presumption of personal agency in behavior and experience, and the dynamic force of fantasy in life experience. Here I am suggesting that the drive model (but not the libido/aggression theory) is the core of an interpretive system that powerfully supports each of these central psychoanalytic assumptions. Let us now see how drive relates to each of them.

Drive and conflict. Because in Freud's dual-instinct theory the drives have incompatible aims, conflict is inherent in psychological life; it is a fundamental characteristic of human nature. Conflict has a very specific meaning in psychoanalytic theory. Like instinct itself, it is pre-experiential, and it is inevitable because of the irreconcilable demands of the two drives. Conflict is not the result of frustration—quite to the contrary, conflict is most likely what causes any experienced frustration. Put another way, conflict is not exclusively interpersonal and does not depend on one person's goals having been thwarted by another person. This is an aspect of what Schafer (1970, 1983) has called Freud's "tragic vision." As in all tragedy, conflict is decreed by fate—in Freud's terminology, it is decreed by our phylogenetic inheritance.

There is some controversy about whether the incompatibility of the drives themselves can be a source of conflict. Otto Fenichel, for one, believed that conflict could originate only in the tension between discharge of some impulse and prohibition of that discharge based on anxiety or guilt. The apparent incompatibility of the drives is deceptive; Fenichel argues that drives having contradictory aims can be satisfied sequentially or, at times, even simultaneously (1945, p. 130). Charles Brenner picks up and endorses this line of argument, writing that drive derivatives are never in conflict just because their aims are different or even if they are logically incompatible (1982, p. 33). For Fenichel and Brenner, conflict essentially reflects the strain between psychic structures.

I believe that this formulation is misleading, and conveys a narrow vision of human conflict. LaPlanche and Pontalis suggest that Freud not only believed in conflict based on the incompatibility of the drives, but thought this to be his most radical explanation of the origin of conflict (1973, p. 360). Freud himself makes the point repeatedly. He writes, for example, of "conflicts arising within the libidinal economy in consequence of our bisexual disposition and conflicts between the erotic and the aggressive instinctual components" (1931, p. 220; also 1930, p. 106). Early on, he suggested that "the irreconcilable . . . demands of the two instincts—the sexual and the egoistic—has made men capable of ever higher achievements" (1912b, p. 190). And later, life itself "would consist in the manifestations of the conflict or interaction between the two classes of instincts" (1923b, p. 259). Each formulation makes clear that for Freud conflict not only precedes but gives shape to experience, particularly relational experience.

Drive and agency. David Rapaport made a great deal of the importance of the drives in protecting people from passive submission to external pressures. He wrote that our innate drive endowment guarantees autonomy from the environment; it provides our ultimate "safeguard from stimulus-response slavery" (1957, p. 727). Rapaport was thinking about drive mainly as a determinant of behavior, but we can take things a step further. The drive theory suggests that not only behavior but human experience itself is shaped by endogenous, pre-experiential needs. On the basis of their unique drive endowment, different people will have different experiences under "objectively" identical stimulus conditions. Environmental factors in development must always be considered in terms of their specific effect on a specific individual. This of course is especially relevant with respect to object relations.

These considerations make it clear that individuals always play an active role in creating their experience—we give what we live through its distinctive shape. The ubiquity of conflict further reflects this, especially from the point of view of the person's behavior. An important implication of conflict theory is that whatever we do, we might always have done something else. However strong a particular motive or tendency might be, there are also motives and tendencies that would be satisfied by a different course of action. The ubiquity of conflict implies the ubiquity of personal choice.

The psychoanalytic vision of agency, of course, must not be confused with any notion of moral or ethical responsibility (Schwartz, 1984). But

it is agency nonetheless. Consider what Freud had to say about personal responsibility for the impulses expressed in dreams:

> Obviously one must hold oneself responsible for the evil impulses of one's dreams. What else is one to do with them? Unless the content of the dream . . . is inspired by alien spirits, it is a part of my own being. If, in defence, I say that what is unknown, unconscious and repressed in me is not my "ego," then I shall not be basing my position upon psycho-analysis, I shall not have accepted its conclusions (1925a, p. 133).

Drive and fantasy. The powerful influence of drive underlies Freud's rationalist vision of psychic reality. Fantasy is the vehicle through which psychic reality gets expressed. It follows that any psychology based in the rationalist tradition will emphasize the importance of fantasy in the dynamics of mental functioning. For Freud, the main significance of fantasy lies in its role as the source of memories that neurotics confused with actual historical (for all intents and purposes, interpersonal) events. Seductions, primal scene experiences, castration threats—each of these may have happened, but because of the power of fantasy it is not necessary to assume they did. In the neuroses (and probably more generally as well) *"it is psychical reality which is the decisive kind"* (Freud, 1916–17, p. 368, original italics).

Authors following Freud have given fantasy an even more encompassing role in the psychic economy. Susan Isaacs clearly states the Kleinian elaboration of his views in her statement, "All impulses, all feelings, all modes of defence are experienced in phantasies which give them *mental* life and show their direction and purpose" (1943, p. 83). Within the tradition of ego psychology, Jacob Arlow has consistently stressed the importance of fantasy as a determinant of all experience, especially of the quality of object relations:

> The type of unconscious fantasy involved determines whether or not the person's body is regarded as a penis or whether the person as a whole is regarded as a breast or, as in the case of narcissistic object choice, whether another person is regarded as a representation of one's own self . . . In [unconscious] fantasies the mental representation of a breast may be *foisted* upon the image of a real external person or, conversely, one's whole body in an unconscious fantasy may be conceived as a representation of one's own or someone else's penis, breast, or feces (1980, p. 114, italics added).

Each of the clinical implications I have described depends on step 2 of Freud's theoretical path—there must be some notion of endogenous mo-

tivational forces that organize human behavior and experience and that may reinforce or oppose each other. None requires the specific interpretive structure imposed by the libido/aggression theory of Freud's third and final step. And, none requires what I consider to be the excesses of Freud's rationalist commitment, the turning away from any serious consideration of external forces in the construction of experience. In the next chapter I will discuss attempts to broaden the interpretive constraints of Freud's thinking by analysts who consider themselves his loyal followers.

Drive Without Meaning

WHEN Freud audaciously proclaimed that a vast spectrum of human achievements—from art to neurosis—arises from conflicted attempts to satisfy elemental, even bestial needs and desires, he captured the world's imagination. Psychoanalytic drive theory gave us an unexpected vision of the passions that move us; it deepened our understanding of both human accomplishment and human suffering. The theory's impact has been felt far beyond the confines of clinical psychoanalysis, reaching into the humanities and the social sciences.

But like all great visions, the drive theory was partial, and both its creator and his disciples expected too much of it. They believed that it would be more than a window into the soul, that it could offer more than a novel, startling glimpse of some powerful disclaimed motives: they expected it to be the last word on the subject of motivation itself, perhaps even on human nature. Today many people still believe that everything Freud invented depends on it. As a result, "drive" has become much more (or much less) than a clinically and theoretically fertile idea; it is a battle cry asserting partisan loyalty.

Partisanship is a two-way street, and the debate over drive theory is usually carried on by those who would preserve it at all costs and those who would get rid of it at all costs. In this chapter I will discuss the strategies of the preservationists. My thesis is this: Beginning shortly after Freud's death, many of his most influential followers became convinced that clinical evidence could not support an interpretive system organized on the vicissitudes of sexual and aggressive urges. They believed that the system was reductionist and too confining clinically. But because so much that was psychoanalytic—even the very idea of "depth psychology"—ap-

peared to depend on the libido/aggression theory, they could not simply turn their backs on the hypothesized role of the drives. So they had to reformulate the drive concept itself.

I will outline five strategies by which these followers of Freud have attempted to retain the term drive or instinctual drive while fundamentally altering its implications. They are roughly divisible into two broad categories. In the first, the focus is on changing the relationship between psychic energy, the mover of the mind, on the one hand, and the specific aims of libido and aggression on the other. The second centers on Freud's rationalist vision of the mind and attempts to derive motives at least in part from interpersonal experience, not only from the workings of endogenous processes.

There are authors who endorse one or more of the strategies while rejecting others. No pattern emerges, which accounts for some of the conceptual confusion that exists in psychoanalytic theory today. Needless to say, the division of various approaches into five strategies is heuristic only. I do not imply any conscious strategizing on the part of the authors involved, nor are the distinctions among the approaches as clear-cut as any attempt at categorization might suggest. I will state the strategies briefly and then discuss them in some detail.

1. The redefinition of drive as an energy without quality. Foreshadowed by Bibring (1936), this strategy is the thrust of Rapaport's writings on the "economic" point of view within psychoanalysis (1959, 1960). Schafer (1968) temporarily adopted this approach, recognizing more clearly than Rapaport how great a departure it is from the original instinct theory.

2. The hypothesis of a third energy source, supplementing the energies derived from sexual and aggressive drives. This is a late idea of Hartmann's (1955) and was endorsed by Loewenstein (1965). In their version, this energy is "noninstinctual"—it is of unspecified quality. In the related but more radical theory of Mahler, it is described as a drive toward individuation (Mahler, Pine, and Bergman, 1975).

3. The postulate of an initial phase of energic undifferentiation. Under this modification of the genetic approach to drive theory, libido and aggression as drive qualities (and thus as determinants of experience) are not present at birth but emerge in the course of the child's development. Fenichel (1945) was the first major proponent of this strategy, and it was developed into widely accepted form by Jacobson (1954, 1964).

4. The definition of drive as representation and the merger of the con-

cepts "drive" and "wish." Within the terms of this strategy, drive no longer aims simply at the relief of tension. Rather, the aim is the creation of situations that have been satisfying at some point in the person's life. The strategy is best known in the writings of Schur (1966) and appears as well in Gill (1963).

5. The explicit integration of environmental factors (especially object relations) into the theory of drive formation. The quality of early experience with others rather than endogenous needs determines the essence of the drives themselves. In different ways this viewpoint has been pursued by Kernberg (1976, 1982) and by Loewald (1969, 1970, 1977).

Energy without quality

One of the first of the many wrenching schisms that have marked the history of psychoanalysis was the defection of Carl Jung. Freud's first recruit from outside Vienna, Jung quickly became both an admirer of Freud's and an original contributor to analytic theory. But despite his enthusiasm for the cause, from the beginning Jung harbored doubts about the role of sexuality as Freud described it. In his second letter to Freud—almost a fan letter in tone—he demurs slightly on one point: "it seems to me that though the genesis of hysteria is predominantly, it is not exclusively, sexual. I take the same view of your sexual theory" (letter 2J, 1906; in McGuire, 1974, pp. 4–5).

Seven years after writing this, Jung's small complaint had evolved into a full-fledged repudiation of Freud's drive theory. Libido, he claimed, is a general life force; sexuality is but one of its manifestations. Libido acquires sexual aims in specific situations, generally in the context of particular object relations. But in broad theoretical terms, Jung insisted, "We want to give the concept of libido the position that really belongs to it, which is a purely energic one" (1913, p. 42).

Although the definition of libido was preserved throughout Freud's lifetime, neither the cause of Jung's dissatisfaction nor his proposed solution ever disappeared. Over time more and more analysts confronted the constraints of the interpretive system embodied in the libido theory. As they did, Jung's proposal gradually (and without acknowledgment) worked its way into the psychoanalytic mainstream, shaping the vision of some nominal supporters of the drive model.

In a classic paper presented as an overview of Freud's own position, Edward Bibring took a position that evokes Jung's early dissent. He began

his argument by defining the drives as "disturbing stimuli" that impinge on the mind. This might warn the reader of a greater apostasy to come. A disturbing stimulus is far from the grand passions of love and hate or life and death that Freud envisioned when he spoke of the forces that drive us. Indeed, Bibring quickly went on to question the original classification of the drives, which he dismissed as "a secondary matter," and concluded that "the instincts were not thought of as directing the whole course of mental events, but only as being sources of energy and causes of excitation" (1936, pp. 125–126). Drive lacks direction, quality, and specific aims; it has none of the characteristics that Freud thought were most crucial.

Bibring's argument was developed by David Rapaport. Of all the psychoanalytic theorists operating within the tradition of American ego psychology, Rapaport is in the paradoxical position of being one of the staunchest defenders of the drive theory and, less obviously, one of its severest critics. The paradox grows from his insistence that, although drive has a special status among human motives, sexuality and aggression are not essential concepts in the theory.

Rapaport placed the drives closer to the center of the psychic economy than Bibring did. One of the assumptions of psychoanalytic theory, he believed, is "the *ultimate determination of all behavior by unconscious drives*" (1959, p. 77). The drives are theoretically crucial because without them there would be nothing within us to resist external pressure—we would be enslaved by environmental demands (1958, p. 726; see also Holt, 1965b). Ego autonomy—personal autonomy, really—depends on some notion of an unconditioned, endogenous drive. Not only the patently maladaptive behaviors that constitute neurosis, but the singular actions that give a cast to our individual lives must be explained by something like the drives.

But there is a difference, Rapaport insists in agreement with Bibring, between drive as a mover of the mind and the particular characteristics that the drives are assumed to have. The libido concept originated in Freud's empirical observations, he points out, and acquired systematic importance only as the prototype of a drive-based theory of motivation. Therefore, Rapaport concludes, "The crucial role attributed to libidinal drives is not a theoretical necessity in this system" (1959, p. 47).

Rapaport offers no specific alternative to the libidinal or aggressive drives; he addresses only the formal characteristics of the motives operating within us. He discusses motives as peremptory, cyclic, selective in their

object, and displaceable without taking any position on what their goals might be (1960, p. 865). Thus, at least indirectly, Rapaport leaves psychoanalytic drive theory where Bibring and even Jung did. Drive is reduced to an energy source without specific direction.

Characteristically, Rapaport presents his position as an attempt to review psychoanalytic theory as it stood at the time of his writing. The impression he conveys is that he is saying just what Freud would have said, if only Freud had the time to summarize his views systematically. Gill and Klein address this style, pointing out that Rapaport "went to extreme lengths to keep his role anonymous and to justify his formulations through the work of others" (1964, p. 14). In doing so, Rapaport adopted a rhetorical tactic similar to Jung's. When Jung redefined libido as energy without quality, he presented his new formulation as only a minor emendation of Freud's views. Freud himself was not impressed. He responded furiously, blasting Jung's suggestion as "nothing else but a pushing into the background of the sexual factor in psycho-analytic theory" (1914b, p. 58).

Rapaport followed Jung's lead. Throughout a lengthy account of the evolution of the drive model he fails to mention that by 1905, when Freud first published his views on a libidinal drive, he had already been basing his clinical work on sexuality for nearly two decades. In fact, it is fair to say that metapsychology itself, what Rapaport calls "the system," was built to house what Freud believed he had discovered about the workings of psychosexuality. This included the inevitable appearance of sexual themes in patients' fantasies; the improvement that followed after the fantasies were made conscious; and, with the evolution of psychoanalytic technique, the ubiquitous emergence of an erotic transference. An analogy may help to clarify the way in which Rapaport distorts the importance of sexuality to Freud. The Taj Mahal was built to enshrine the body of a woman. Her body is not an essential part of the structure of the monument. But saying that hardly accounts for its importance in the general picture because, without the body, there would have been no monument. Rapaport's desexualization of drive theory undermines Freud's fundamental intention, because it robs the theory of its interpretive thrust.

Some psychoanalysts have always bristled at the interpretive limitations of the libido theory. Despite very different sensibilities, these authors agree that sexual and aggressive needs cannot fuel all mental activity. Defining drive as an energy without quality—an energy without aims that are innately fixed and that operate pre-experientially—has been one theoretical

path to broadening the theory. Doing so gives the clinical psychoanalyst new interpretive latitude; there is no longer any theoretical necessity to find the sexual or aggressive meanings in all mental acts. There is, of course, no theoretical warrant for doing so either.

A Third Energy Source

There were some early attempts to broaden the interpretive focus of drive theory in Freud's own work and in the work of others while he was still alive. With the advent of the structural model (1923a), forces other than the drives acquired increasing weight in the economy of the mental apparatus. The ego, guided by adaptive and self-preservative needs, is the most prominent of these. Although at first Freud depicted it as the relatively powerless rider of the horse id, this vision quickly gave way to one in which the ego played a decisive role in shaping mental life. The revised anxiety theory (Freud, 1926), Robert Waelder's principle of multiple function (1930), Herman Nunberg's synthetic function of the ego (1930), and Anna Freud's approach to the ego through its defense mechanisms (1936) all contributed to this trend. Each of these new formulations implied the existence of motives that could be decisive in determining behavior but that were not actually derived from the workings of drive.

The genetic point of view, however, saved the unique status of drive in the system even with these new ingredients of the theoretical mix. There were new forces to contend with in understanding experience analytically—but ultimately all of them arose in the life history of the individual as transformations of the original drive endowment. The ego is, after all, merely a specialized (and superficial) layer of the id. Human development itself is the process of creating psychic structure out of the seething cauldron of primitive need.

This changed, however, and drive lost its exclusive motivational role with Heinz Hartmann's concepts of the undifferentiated matrix from which ego and id emerge and of the autonomous functions of the ego (1939a, 1950). Now, for the first time within the mainstream of Freudian psychoanalysis, there were acknowledged psychological functions that could not be explained, even genetically, on the basis of drives. These included adaptive (not psychopathological) behaviors and the adaptive aspects of all (even psychopathological) behaviors.

Although it vitiated the power of the drives, Hartmann's approach did

little to change the nature of the drive concept itself. The new theoretical developments, Rapaport said, made it difficult to maintain that the drives cause all mental activity. But still, he claimed, they "retain a special position in the system of the theory" (1959, p. 68n). The impact of Hartmann's work was similar to what happens when a nation loses part, but not all, of its territory as the result of invasion. The conquered territory might have to submit to a new form of government, but the situation in the unconquered part would remain unchanged. The concept of ego autonomy certainly changed aspects of the explanatory system of psychoanalysis (the analogy holds well because these aspects had been on the periphery of the theory before Hartmann), but it leaves Freud's approach to drive untouched at the core.

Despite its power, and despite Hartmann's tempting suggestion that psychoanalysis could become a general psychology, his early contributions contained an important inconsistency. Hartmann accepted the fundamental Freudian assumption that mind is an energized structure. Any ego function that is not fueled by the drives has, by psychoanalytic fiat, no source of energy at all. What could fuel the workings of the autonomous ego?

Some authors have attempted to locate an energy source in Freud's own drive theory. Rapaport (1960), Robert Holt (1962), and Merton Gill (1963) find references to a noninstinctual energy in the early concepts of "mobile cathectic energy" deployed by the preconscious (system Pcs.) and of "hypercathexis," which explains how a preconscious idea becomes conscious. But these are ideas that Freud proposed in chapter 7 of *The Interpretation of Dreams* (1900). They predate the drive model itself and cannot represent an alternative to instinctual energy. Rapaport, Holt, and Gill were trapped by their zeal to minimize the extent to which the idea of ego autonomy violates the premises of drive theory. Since there is no instinct in *The Interpretation of Dreams*, there is no referent in any contemporary sense for the concept of instinctual energy; and noninstinctual or neutral energy could have had no meaning in 1900.

There is an interesting extension of this line of thought in Gill's interpretation of an important passage in *The Ego and the Id*. Gill holds that Freud's monograph "did introduce a major concept concerning [the] condition of energy: the concept of neutral displaceable energy . . . This 'neutral' energy is in fact described as *neutralized* energy" (1963, p. 42). Gill goes on to quote the passage in which Freud ascribes neutral displaceable energy to "the narcissistic store of libido—that it is desexualized Eros"

(1923a, p. 44). Freud is referring to a quantity of energy, originally instinctual, that has lost its primordial qualities. Gill disregards this crucial genetic point, blurring the concepts "neutral" and "neutralized." This allows a reading of Freud in which the drives lose their unique position as determinants of mental activity—it makes the third-drive strategy of Hartmann seem less radical in its implications. Neutral*ized* energy originates in the drives; neutral energy does not.

Eventually Hartmann was willing to address the radical implications of ego autonomy. He was fully aware of the need to introduce a new source of energy to account for the autonomous functions. And he also knew just how challenging this would be to existing theory, especially to the central assumption that *drive* is a demand made on the mind for work. Accordingly, he moved cautiously toward the hypothesis of an energy source independent of the two drives (see especially Hartmann, 1948, 1950, 1953; Hartmann, Kris, and Loewenstein, 1949).

The problem is not mentioned in *Ego Psychology and the Problem of Adaptation,* although the concept of the undifferentiated matrix apparently demands it, and was not addressed at all in the decade following its publication. Hartmann's first solution was to rely on the idea of neutralization (1950), basing his approach on a reading of Freud's concept of sublimation similar to Gill's. But he saw that neutralization is not up to the theoretical task. Because it refers to the modification of instinctual energy, it cannot operate *ab initio* and is incapable of explaining the energizing of *primarily* autonomous functions. A third energy source, independent of the drives from the beginning, is needed.

Hartmann's final position is contained in an unelaborated footnote to his late paper "Notes on the Theory of Sublimation." There, in a passage referring to the origin of energy, he states: "A terminological note is to the point here. Strictly speaking, energy that from the start belongs to the ego can, of course, not be termed 'deinstinctualized' or 'neutralized.' It could be called 'noninstinctual' and probably is best called 'primary ego energy'" (1955, p. 240n).

Note Hartmann's caution, his unwillingness to call a spade a spade. What he has done goes to the heart of the interpretive system of psychoanalysis: he has rejected the assumption that all motives originate in sexual and aggressive needs. Since there is a primary ego energy, some behaviors and experiences are not organized around libidinal or destructive needs. Hartmann is whistling past a theoretical graveyard when he dismisses this new idea as a "terminological note."

Neither Hartmann nor his closest collaborators attempted to describe the qualities that a third energy source might have. In the work of Ernst Kris (1955), Rapaport (1959), and Rudolph Loewenstein (1965), non-instinctual energy is presumed to fuel mental events that are neither dynamically nor genetically related to sexuality or aggression. In Freud's drive theory there simply are no such mental events. Hartmann's third energy source broadens the theory of psychoanalysis much as the strategy of energy without quality does, by introducing a large area of motivational indeterminacy. For Hartmann, it isn't that all drive lacks direction, but that some drive does. This hands over to clinical inquiry what had been laid out specifically by the metapsychology.

Although Hartmann never suggested a direction for his third energy source, Margaret Mahler did. In an early formulation, she characterized this force as a drive toward separation (Mahler and Gosliner, 1955). Later she revised her views, proposing that the primary drive is directed toward individuation, with separation merely one subsidiary aspect of the process (Mahler, Pine, and Bergman, 1975). This is an example of Mahler's overall theoretical strategy of particularizing (and personalizing) Hartmann's broadly sketched principles.

Initial Energic Undifferentiation

Simply stripping drive of its quality or adding a third energy source does not address all the problems of the libido/aggression theory. Although they have the potential for broadening the theory's interpretive implications, these strategies leave Freud's rationalism untouched. The mind is still energized—driven—exclusively by internal forces, and those forces themselves are shaped by phylogeny and not at all by experience. But even for some loyal Freudians the residue of life experience must be integrated into the motivational system of psychoanalysis at its most fundamental level.

There have been three strategies for accomplishing this goal, which can be arrayed on a continuum from less to more radical. I will begin with the first, the "strategy of initial energic undifferentiation." The essential premise of this strategy is that libido and aggression are maturational or developmental derivatives of a psychic energy that at the origin of life has no specific quality. In its initial state of undifferentiation, drive looks something like Rapaport's energy without quality, but the implications of this strategy are more radical.

The idea is generally introduced by its supporters as a refinement of the

drive model. It is needed, these authors suggest, because of some problems that arise in understanding the nature of drive operations in the earliest days of life. Because it is presented so cautiously, undifferentiation can easily look like a kind of technical nicety, an arcane theoretical wrinkle relevant only to the very beginnings of infancy. It can be hard to ferret out its clinical implications for work with adult patients, but they are there, and they are profound. Followed to its logical conclusions, the hypothesis provides a strong and clearly stated alternative to the interpretive system of the drive model.

The concept of undifferentiation was foreshadowed in Otto Fenichel's 1935 critique of the death instinct and first articulated by him ten years later. At the beginning of life, the infant's aim is to incorporate its objects. This simultaneously brings it close to them and destroys them. The two effects of incorporation—and the infant's desires themselves—are for all intents and purposes indistinguishable. Fenichel writes that "in these early periods libidinal and aggressive tendencies are so interwoven that they never can be entirely separated from each other; it seems as if these stages represent an integrated state, from which, later, eros and aggression are differentiated; only later do love and hate develop as opposite qualities" (1945, p. 60).

The idea of undifferentiated energy was developed by Edith Jacobson, and it continues to be most closely associated with her work. In her 1954 paper and her 1964 book, both entitled "The Self and the Object World," she addressed a number of problems in applying drive theory to the earliest phase of infancy. The most serious problem was the assumption that at the beginning aggression (like libido) must be directed inward; its object must be the self. The theory suggests no way in which this self-directed destructiveness could be modulated either by neutralization or by fusion with libido at this stage of life. The neonate would destroy itself, using as a weapon some sort of psychosomatic attack. Although it is a logical implication of the theory, this prediction accords poorly with anything about infants that we can observe.

Jacobson concluded that there must be no such thing as pure aggression (or pure libido) so early on. Instead, "at the very beginning of life, the instinctual energy is still in an undifferentiated state . . . from birth on it develops into two kinds of psychic drives with different qualities under the influence of external stimulations, of psychic growth and the opening up and increasing maturation of pathways for outside discharge" (1964, p. 13).

Jacobson's hypothesis has been widely accepted by analysts asserting

loyalty to Freud's drive model. Prominent among these authors are Max Schur (1958, 1966), Margaret Mahler (Mahler and Gosliner, 1955), and Rudolph Loewenstein (1965). Loewenstein, bridging the gap between Jacobson and Hartmann, extended the concept of undifferentiated energy to make it the source not only of libido and aggression but of a noninstinctual ego energy as well.

The most radical implications of the hypothesis hinge on what may appear to be an obscure point: how does energic differentiation occur? The theoretical problems to which Fenichel and Jacobson addressed the concept could be served simply by the idea of a maturational unfolding of libidinal and aggressive drives, along the lines of the endogenously determined progressive appearance of libidinal phases. But authors working with the phase of undifferentiation have a more ambitious project in mind.

Consider Jacobson's clearest statement on the issue: "With birth . . . pleasurable and unpleasurable sensations begin to be perceived and become attached to, though still confused with, beginning outside perceptions. Energic differentiation occurs; libidinal and aggressive cathectic gathering poles are formed around nuclei of as yet unorganized and disconnected memory traces" (1964, p. 52). A "cathectic gathering pole" (it is hard to imagine anyone who really wanted to clarify things inventing such a term) is simply a collection of emotionally similar interpersonal situations. These cluster together in memory and become forged into homogeneous mental representations. In turn, the representations "attract" undifferentiated energy. The energy attracted to the "pleasurable" situations becomes libido; that which is attracted to the unpleasurable situations becomes aggression.

The strategy of initial energic differentiation represents a bridge between strategies which strip the quality from drive and those which more radically attack Freud's rationalism. Jacobson's undifferentiated energy in infants functions as a life force that evokes Jung's definition of libido. But the drives of older children and adult patients are differentiated. These of course are the drives that are of greatest interest to clinical psychoanalysts, and they have a specific direction, significantly determined by the events of the individual's life history. Differentiation depends on the felt quality of early experience; the drives are no longer entirely endogenously shaped and pre-experiential.

In advancing her formulation, Jacobson expressed awareness of how close she was to providing a dichotomous alternative to classical drive theory. She wrote: "While such a conception may be reminiscent of the

frustration-aggression theory, it should be noted that the transformation of undifferentiated psychophysiological energy into two qualitatively different kinds of psychic drives is here regarded as psychobiologically predetermined and as promoted by internal maturational factors *as well as by* external stimuli" (1964, p. 14, my italics). Jacobson is trying to bring psychobiology and maturation to the rescue of a tattered theory. She suggests that energic differentiation will happen regardless of the child's idiosyncratic experience; it is fated, regardless of what occurs. But the statement is dictated more by loyalty than by the force of logic. Jacobson is concerned that she has shifted the focus of Freud's approach: rather than drive endowment shaping experience with others, experience with others has become a crucial (and conceptually inseparable) determinant of what appears in the adult as drive endowment.

Consider how Mahler applied Jacobson's point of view, giving the idea of cathectic gathering poles an experiential and even human face. Libido and aggression develop out of the initial undifferentiated energy when the infant is able to distinguish between "'good' and 'bad'. . . images of mother and self" (Mahler and Gosliner, 1955, p. 198). With this, Mahler makes it clear that there is a relationship with the mother, and that it has experiential qualities (it is either "good" or "bad") before there is either libido or aggression. To put this in its baldest terms, for both Mahler and Jacobson there is a relationship before there is a drive. Further, the nature of the relationship has at least some influence on the characteristic of the drive itself.

Drive or Wish?

The other radical attempts to escape the constraints of Freud's rationalism go to the core of the definition of drive itself. The first, less drastic approach builds on an ambiguity in Freud's many discussions of drive. In his introduction to "Instincts and their Vicissitudes," James Strachey (1957) notes that sometimes Freud spoke of drive as the *mental representative* of an internal stimulus (1905a, 1911b, 1915a). But he also spoke of drive as the somatic stimulus itself, so that the additional concept of an *instinctual representative* was necessary to account for its effect on the psychic apparatus (1915b, 1915c).

Strachey concluded that the contradiction is less significant than it appears to be. Drive is inherently ambiguous, he said, because of Freud's determined effort to locate it on the conceptual frontier between mind and

body (1957, p. 113). Strachey was able to minimize the apparent inconsistency because he made an important (and in my opinion correct) assumption about what Freud thought needed to be represented—what it is about a drive that becomes mental. He assumed that what becomes mental is a *need,* a feeling of tension that demands relief.

On Strachey's reading, it matters little whether we define drive as the somatic changes that give rise to the felt need or as the feeling of need itself. What is crucial for Freud's drive theory is that what is represented initially is simply a need and not a need *for* something. Life's accidents (borrowing Freud's term) sooner or later provide something suited to satisfy the need, and that something achieves the status of *object.* Freud stressed this in his definition: "The object . . . is what is most variable about an instinct and is not originally connected with it" (1915a, p. 122).

A number of authors working within the classical psychoanalytic tradition have built on the ambiguity noted by Strachey to effect their own redefinition of drive and their own recasting of drive theory. This strategy hinges on a distortion of Freud's ideas about what is represented in the mental representation of a drive: the theorists using it assume that not only the need but also a source of satisfaction are necessary aspects of the representation. Understood this way, the drive itself does not simply reflect the flow of an inner force; it is intrinsically shaped by experience.

The primary exponent of this strategy has been Max Schur. At birth, Schur suggests, there are no drives; there are only somatic needs that must be met for the sake of preserving a homeostatic balance. Neither is there a mind in any recognizable sense during these earliest days; the neonate is equipped only with a simple reflex apparatus capable of discharging the tension of need. With maturation, the infant becomes capable of mentally representing the stimuli that arise within his body. At that point we can speak meaningfully both of a mind and of instinctual drives. Therefore, Schur concludes, the definition of drive includes "perceptions and memory traces" (1966, p. 69). The id, as seat of the drives, is "structured," so that it includes these ideational contents.

Freud realized that drive needs become associated with perceptions and memory traces. We remember inner states, he often said: the tension that accompanies a surge of need, the pleasure that accompanies discharge. But Schur goes far beyond this. We remember not only what satisfaction felt like, he says, but also the circumstances associated with the rise of tensions and with the ways in which the needs were met. Accordingly, what is mentally represented by drive as Schur redefines it is not simply need, but rather the entire history of the flow of need and its satisfaction.

A similar approach underlies Gill's view of the id. Gill agrees with Schur that the definition of drive as a representation means that there must be ideas built into the drives themselves. The unconscious, and the id too, is the container of these ideas as well as of inchoate instinctual urges (1963, p. 134). The id as well as the ego has an inherent relationship to external reality, and even obeys the laws of the secondary process (pp. 146–147).

Notice that, as Schur and Gill put things, drives do not exist at the beginning of life, but only needs, acted upon reflexively by a prepsychological organism. We can speak of drives only when the infant has already accumulated some experience of the world, when he has some mental image of the conditions in which the need has been met. The drive does not simply aim at removing the tension of need. Instead it aims at creating a particular situation—typically, and despite the measured vagueness of Schur's and Gill's language, an interpersonal situation—in which the need can be satisfied.

There is a well-established psychoanalytic construct that covers the ground described by Schur and Gill. It is the wish, the central concept of Freud's motivational system prior to his introduction of the drive model. Wishes are desires to recreate situations in which some important need has been satisfactorily met. But Freud made it clear that there may be wishes for anything that a person might want at one time or another. The wish might be for a situation that permits sexual expression, or for one that feels safe, or for one that encourages feelings of competence, or for anything else. The emphasis, always, is on circumstances—on context.

There are no specific needs assumed to lie behind the wish: "The wish model gives us great latitude of interpretive possibility; we are quite free to fill in the need which the wish is designed to satisfy" (Greenberg and Mitchell, 1983, p. 29). The conceptual role of drive theory is to fill in the indeterminacy of the wish model. The direction attributed to the drives defines the irreducible content of wishes. Drive is the construct that points the way for the practicing analyst attempting to gain entry into the nature of what is wished for.

These considerations clarify the problems involved in redefining drives as representations. Drive may (as Strachey allows) represent an endogenous need. But it does not represent the situations in which the need has been satisfied; that precisely defines the distinction between drive and wish. *The wish represents situations; the drive specifies the need that the situation must satisfy.* The distinction is especially important in understanding Freud's rationalist approach to the problem of object relations. Objects are an integral and established part of the wish, but they are a creation of

the drive. To put it another way, the object precedes the wish, but the drive precedes the object. In moving beyond the wish model to the theory of instinctual drive, Freud replaced a vision of motivation based in the tendency to recreate past experiences with a vision of motivation that is pre-experiential.

I will later argue (in Chapter 7 especially) that there is great clinical and theoretical value in assuming that the fundamental motivational unit of psychoanalysis must include some experiential determinants. But the assumption does violate the premises of Freud's drive model. Drives that include representational components are not drives at all; they are wishes. In their redefinition of drive as representation, Gill and Schur have blurred the distinction between drive and wish. This becomes explicit in two statements derived from their approach. Peter Wolff writes that "the infant having no mental representation does not have an instinctual drive in a psychoanalytic sense; there can be no wishes without such representation" (cited in Panel, 1968, p. 622). And Charles Fisher makes the same point: "we cannot speak of instinctual drives until psychic structure develops, until the formation of the 'wish,' that is, when memory traces of experiences of gratification and frustration are laid down" (1965, p. 273). Schur, Gill, and their many followers have retained the term "drive" while discarding the concept.*

Experience and Drive

Of the five strategies I am considering, this one has the most radical implications for the interpretive system of psychoanalysis. The attempt to integrate experience into the structure of drive turns Freud's model on its head. The approach is derivative of but much more far-reaching than the strategies of initial energic undifferentiation and drive as representation. Here there is no pretense of any pre-experiential (biological or otherwise) component of drive. Aggression and libido are motivational systems that emerge from the matrix of early object relations—especially from the relationship between mother and infant.

---

*Joseph Sandler has undertaken a major revision of psychoanalytic theory shaped largely by his reliance on the wish rather than the drive as the fundamental motivational unit (see, for example, Sandler and Sandler, 1978). Sandler is clear that the wish may be for a situation that permits the discharge of sexual or aggressive tensions (which he still calls "drives"), but that it also may be for something else. Holt (1976) argued for a shift from drive to wish along similar lines. These authors distinguish between the two concepts rather than blending them together.

The two most important proponents of this strategy are Hans Loewald and Otto Kernberg. Despite vastly different sensibilities in other areas of their psychoanalytic thinking, with respect to the organization and development of drive Loewald and Kernberg have arrived at compatible views. Even in this area, however, their approaches are sufficiently different to require that we examine them separately.

Loewald uses language that appears to keep him well within the classical model. Instinct (a term he prefers to the more commonly used "drive") is "the most primitive element or unit of motivation" (1971, p. 119). And, he suggests, even with the development and increasing influence of higher level psychic organization and structure, "instincts as the original motive forces never become extinct" (p. 112). Both comments are perfectly at home in Freud's thinking.

But even from the beginning there was something peculiar about the drives as he envisioned them. In his early work Loewald built upon but went beyond Freud's 1920 concept of Eros and Hartmann's theory of adaptation. For Hartmann, the ego is a specific organ of adaptation, required in humans because the drives are inherently alienated from reality (1939a). Loewald rejects this formulation; in his view, the *person* is innately adapted, connected with the interpersonal surround from the very beginning of life. The difference between id and ego is not the difference between blind need and socially mediated restrictions, or between the pleasure and reality principles. The two structures reflect alternative, developmentally changing modes of living in the real world, with other people. Thus Loewald concludes that "instinctual drives are as primarily related to 'objects,' to the external world, as the ego is" (1960, p. 235).

The formulation is aesthetically and clinically compelling, but it certainly distorts the theory on which it is nominally based. For Loewald, the drives have an immediate relationship to the object world. This idea has much in common with the views of Melanie Klein and Fairbairn. But it stands in sharp contradistinction to the theories of both Freud and Hartmann, who see object relatedness—especially relatedness to an external, non-autoerotic object—as a crucial and difficult developmental achievement.

For a decade Loewald ignored the crucial question of how his "most primitive unit of motivation" comes into being. Within the terms of classical drive theory as I have described it, this is a nonquestion. Freud took the position that somatic changes at the anatomical source give rise to tensions that impinge on the mind: these are the "most primitive units." Drive theorists who reject the somatic origin of the drives cannot rely on

this explanation—they must insist that the urges that become shaped into motives simply arise, automatically, according to some rhythm that is part and parcel of being human. In either case, some increases in tension may be stimulated—physiologically or psychologically—by an external agency, but this is "accidental" and simply changes the timing of what would have happened sooner or later anyway.

Loewald eventually took a strong position on the origin of the drive impulse, and in a way that left Freud's theory far behind. Acknowledging that he has changed Freud's definition of instinct, he writes:

> instinctual drives in their original form are not forces immanent in an autonomous, separate primitive psyche, but are resultants of tensions within the mother-child psychic matrix and later between the immature infantile psyche and the mother. Instincts, in other words, are to be seen as relational phenomena from the beginning and not as autochthonous forces seeking discharge (1969, pp. 321–322).

A year later Loewald returned to the problem, taking an even stronger position. The drives are given their very shape by the child's earliest social relationships:

> instinctual drives, as psychic forces, are processes taking place within a field— the mother-infant psychic matrix; and that their character as instincts as well as the character of the emerging individual psyche are determined by the changing characteristics of that matrix-field (1970, p. 291).

Although they are internalized as a result of what Loewald calls "narcissistic transformation," the drives "never relinquish their character as relational phenomena" (1970, p. 292; also Loewald, 1971, 1977). Moreover, the drives themselves continue to be modified by "present psychic fields of which the individual has become a relatively autonomous constituent" (1970, p. 292). The shaping of drive by interpersonal experience is not a one-time thing but continues throughout life.

It follows, and Loewald makes it explicit, that the drives are no longer innate phylogenetic needs. Further, they are not the crucial determinants that color perceptions but rather are themselves forged from perceptions. Building on the strategy of drive as representation, he radically alters the approach to object relations: "the object does not become 'assigned' to the instinct . . . but contributes crucially to the organization of instincts qua instincts, just as instinctual forces crucially contribute to the organization of objects qua objects" (1971, p. 130).

This formulation goes considerably beyond Loewald's earlier view that

drives are simply object-related from the beginning; he has arrived at an approach to drive that was unique in psychoanalytic theory when he proposed it. To summarize: The infant is born with certain biologically determined needs—essentially those involved in the maintenance of physiological equilibrium. These are not yet drives because they have no representational component and therefore lack status as psychological phenomena. Moreover, the infant is unable to distinguish these needs as his own because of his cognitive inability to differentiate self from object.

The infant's earliest needs acquire psychological meaning only in the context of his relationship with his mother. The mother's ministrations, in addition to meeting the biological needs, also bring organization to them. Her higher-level abilities to understand, categorize, and form a mental image of the needs is an important aspect of her caretaking role. These abilities in turn help the infant to organize and represent his needs, always in the context of the dyadic relationship. *Inchoate need becomes drive in the context of and as a result of this organizing process.* Need becomes separated from response so that drive and object emerge, developmentally, as more or less autonomous representations.

Loewald believes that the organization of need which occurs in the early relationship with the mother leads to the emergence of two independent motivational systems that can be labeled, consistent with Freud's later dual-instinct theory, libido and aggression. The reason for taking this final step, however, is unclear at best. Why should only two instincts emerge out of the mother-infant dyad? How does it happen that the motives emerging out of a social bond happen to be the same as the motives that Freud believed were handed down phylogenetically? And since for Loewald the process begins with particular dyads, why should the motives have any universal quality? These questions cannot be answered within the developmental framework Loewald has provided.

OTTO Kernberg's approach to the problem of drive has a long and complex history, which is significantly determined by the tension between his efforts to create a unique "object relations" theory and his interest in remaining within the framework of ego psychology as delineated by Mahler and Jacobson.* His writings, therefore, are paradoxical. On the one hand,

---

*Here I concentrate only on Kernberg's two latest versions of his drive theory. A full account of the evolution of his thinking is available in Greenberg and Mitchell (1983). See also Mitchell (1981); Klein and Tribich (1981).

he is a trenchant critic of authors, such as Fairbairn and Kohut, who have rejected drive theory (Kernberg, 1980, 1982). On the other hand, he overturns Freud by integrating experience into the structure of drive.

Drive is no longer an irreducible stimulus arising from the body and impinging on the mind. It is not even the "most primitive unit of motivation" that it is for Loewald. Rather, Kernberg's drive is a motivational system that is itself constructed out of "building blocks." These building blocks are the "internalization units" that also form the constituents of the tripartite psychic structure: they consist of a representations of the self and an object in relationship to each other, along with an affective valence that gives the represented relationship its particular emotional tone.

The elementary units in Kernberg's system, the building blocks, are object relations that have achieved internal representation. Freud's rationalism is nowhere in sight. There is a vestige of internal determinants of experience in the affective tone that colors the representations (and colored the original interactions). A particular exchange between two people (mother and infant being the earliest and most significant case in point) will not be encoded by the infant as good or bad simply on the basis of whether it was "objectively" satisfying. Equally important is the infant's particular affective state at the time of the interaction. Affects themselves are irreducible in Kernberg's system. They are also both the earliest and throughout life the primary motivational system (1982, p. 907). Affects are for Kernberg what instincts are for Loewald.

Kernberg relies on a systems approach to explain the relationship of libido and aggression to the fundamental internalization units. Basically, libido is the motivational system that derives from accumulated good experiences, aggression is the system that integrates and expresses bad experiences. Kernberg writes:

> instincts in the human being *develop gradually* out of the assembly of these "building blocks," so that the series of pleasurable affect-determined units and the series of unpleasurable affect-determined units gradually evolve into the libidinally invested and aggressively invested constellations of psychic drive systems—that is, into libido and aggression, respectively, as the two major psychological drives (1976, p. 87, my italics).

Giving his hypothesis a more personal cast, Kernberg eventually suggested: "Love and hate . . . become stable intrapsychic structures, in genetic continuity through various developmental stages, and, by that very continuity, consolidate into libido and aggression" (1982, p. 908). With

this he reverses Freud's thoughts on drive and object relations. For Freud, love and hate are transformations of drive-derived impulses and differ from those impulses on two counts. First, they are feelings that one person has for another; they express, as Freud said, "the relations of the *total ego* to objects" (1915a, p. 137). Second, they are feelings that temporally outlast the impulses, so that we feel love or hate even when the sexual or aggressive drive has been satiated (1921). For Kernberg, the relationship is primary, the drive derivative.

We see in these formulations an echo of Jacobson's undifferentiated energy attracted to cathectic gathering poles and bifurcating into libido and aggression, but there is no longer any bow to biological or other internal determinants. For Jacobson, the early experiences merely channeled the flow of energy, which was still conceived as a biological product. Here the components of the drives—the very stuff of which they are made—are the early relational experiences.

Comparing Kernberg's views with Loewald's, what is most important is a point of agreement: both authors construe drive as a motivational system that emerges from the earliest social experiences. The influence of these experiences is expressed in Loewald's language in terms of the mother's organization of the child's inchoate needs; for Kernberg, the represented experiences of loving and hating become the building blocks of the needs themselves.

Two important differences between Kernberg's and Loewald's views deserve mention. First, for Loewald, both drive and object emerge from a kind of undifferentiated matrix. For Kernberg, the object is clearly present before the drive is formed—in fact, it is possible and even necessary to talk about object-directed emotions before the appearance of libido and aggression. Second, Loewald, because of his consistent stress on the initial state of undifferentiation, has no framework for encompassing the child's role in coloring the nature of her original experience. Kernberg has such a framework in his concept of affect as an irreducible, endogenous determinant of the nature of the interaction. But affect is not drive, and libido and aggression have no fundamental theoretical role in Kernberg's system.

Revised Drives and Clinical Inquiry

With characteristic clarity, Charles Brenner has given voice to a question expressed less straightforwardly by many theorists: "What one must decide, if one is to introduce real change into psychoanalytic theory, is

whether one thinks it unjustified to generalize about conscious and unconscious wishes as Freud did, by dividing them into two groups, libidinal and aggressive" (1980a, p. 211). Increasingly, even analysts who identify themselves as classical Freudians are answering Brenner's question in the negative. There is a burgeoning consensus that deriving all wishes from the workings of hypothesized libidinal and aggressive drives is no longer justified. I would say that this opinion is held so widely that the libido/aggression theory as an interpretive system no longer exists, certainly not in the sense that Freud (and Brenner) had in mind.

In the last chapter I suggested that four characteristics define drive as the interpretive system of psychoanalysis. As modified by the strategies outlined in this chapter, none of these characteristics remains intact.

Drive is a demand made on the mind for work. It is the only source of the energy that fuels the operations of the mind. Although each of the Freudian theorists arrives at a different conclusion, there is unanimous agreement that libido and aggression are *not* the only movers of the mind. There are third drives with unspecified direction in Hartmann's work, and independent drives toward individuation in Mahler's. There is undifferentiated energy, which in Jacobson's version of things continues to fuel some mental activities throughout life. There are wishes, which aim at reestablishing situations rather than at discharging tensions, in the formulation of Schur.

These changes introduce, quite deliberately, areas of indeterminacy that broaden the interpretive system of psychoanalysis. Any particular behavior, or any experience, may be driven by sexual or aggressive impulses. But, equally, the motive may be something quite different. Consider two comments from important theorists who, at the time the comments were written were considered as operating comfortably within the drive model. The first is from Fenichel: "all defense is 'relative defense'; relative to one layer it is defense, and at the same time, relative to another layer it is that which is warded off" (1941, p. 62). Gill puts the matter even more strongly: "In general, a behavior is a defense in relation to a drive more primitive than itself, and a drive in relation to a defense more advanced than itself" (1963, pp. 122–123).

These formulations answer Brenner's question. If anything can be a drive, then not everything can be derived from the libidinal or aggressive urge. The concept of drive itself loses a great deal of its meaning; certainly it cannot guide psychoanalytic inquiry in the way that Freud intended.

Drive is no longer the Rosetta Stone that Ogden (1984) argues it once was and that Brenner hopes it still can be.

Clinically, these modifications of the drive theory lead to new ways of constructing the meaning that patients attach to their experiences, especially to their relationships. There is a nice example of this in a paper of Loewenstein's. Here Loewenstein argues for retaining libido as a drive but for replacing aggression with a version of the self-preservative instincts. He was trying to maintain a dualistic framework, but could no longer accept the direction of the drives as Freud had defined it. Loewenstein describes the experience of a female patient:

> She remembered having, as a child, established a complete hierarchy, beginning at the bottom with her small brother and rising through her sister, herself and her mother successively up to her father. This hierarchy was founded upon various considerations, one of them being moral power and another sexual knowledge. Can we not discern here . . . a sexual hierarchy based upon dominance—a dominance which determines sexual behavior? In my patient this hierarchy based upon dominance was cut across by a hierarchy based upon the possession of a penis, for the two hierarchies did not by any means coincide (1940, pp. 390–391).

Loewenstein makes it clear that his patient's childhood experience was significantly shaped by her developmental needs, and that these needs themselves were based in her drive endowment. She did not simply observe a hierarchy that existed independently within the family structure— she "established" (that is, created) it. This is a powerful example of how the rationalist sensibility of drive theory works.

But without libido and aggression as the fundamental interpretive principles of psychoanalysis, the constructed hierarchies look different than they would have to Freud. Having redefined the drives, Loewenstein understands the patient's perception of her family as organized around sex (possession of a penis) and self-preservation (possession of power and knowledge). He makes the point explicit: "We have here a combination of two sets of factors, sexual and self-preservative, each of which in turn may come to the top" (p. 391).

Drive has a qualitatively specific nature—an inherent direction—that determines its aims. This principle is decisively undercut with the reformulations of drive. Rapaport's energy without quality, Hartmann's noninstinctual energy, and Jacobson's undifferentiated energy have no stated quality—

they pointedly lack direction. Each is a source of energy, but unlike libido and aggression they have no specifiable aims. Wishes cannot be reduced to sexual or aggressive aims; the wish generally defies reductionism. This undermines the determined dualism that was a critical aspect of Freud's model.

Dualism was the foundation of the psychoanalytic assumption that conflict lies behind virtually all mental activity. Freud found conflict at every level of psychological analysis (he discusses motivational, defensive, interpersonal, and societal conflicts). So he built a theory in which conflict is ubiquitous, from the bottom up; in his late theory it was built into the structure of every living cell. Because the two drives inherently oppose each other, conflict itself is pre-experiential. This is an essential aspect of what Schafer (1970) has called the "tragic vision" of psychoanalysis.

What happens when drive has been redefined? Without the specificity of Freud's model—without the presumed opposition of the drives—there can be no support for his radical vision of conflict. Consider how two of the revisionists whose work I have been discussing, Rapaport and Fenichel, were obliged to reformulate conflict.

Rapaport saw the implications of his redefinition of drive as energy without quality. Since there is no inherent direction to drive, there can be no conflict between incompatible drives. But Rapaport, like Freud, was committed to a rationalist view of mind; conflict had to originate internally and pre-experientially. As a result, he is left with this:

> the motor, perceptual, and memory apparatuses, as well as other inborn apparatuses such as those of affect expression, stimulus barrier, etc., have definite thresholds which are their *structural characteristics*. These *structural characteristics* will set limits to the discharge of drive tension, that is, to the pleasure principle, even when the need-satisfying object is present, and even before drive discharge is prevented by the absence of the need-satisfying object. The very nature of structure will always prevent total discharge of tension (1951, pp. 362–363).

This is a vision of conflict based entirely on the nature of a mechanism, on the distinction between energy and structure. The mind is a machine, and its ability to discharge tensions is limited, much as friction saps mechanical energy or wire impedes the flow of electricity.

Because he stripped drive of its direction, Rapaport arrived at a vision of conflict without conflicting motives. Conflict originates neither in love and hate nor in unfulfilled desire. There is nothing of the grand clash of

passions we find in Freud, nothing of the battle between the individual and society that characterizes Freud's late, pessimistic vision of man's fate—because there is nothing inherent in human nature that would be socially intolerable. Rescuing the theory from its narrowness, Rapaport impoverishes it clinically.

Fenichel was more radical when he approached the problem. We see conflicts between opposing instinctual tendencies, he observed, but the theory of undifferentiated energy undercuts the assumption that these reflect "a genuine and unconditioned dichotomy, operative from the very beginning" (1945, pp. 60–61). Conflict is not, as it was for Freud, the inevitable result of our fundamentally divided human nature.

This sets a new clinical task for the analyst. Fenichel suggests that "conflicts have a history; they came into being at a certain point of development and remain conflicts only as long as certain conditions prevail" (p. 60). The focus of analytic inquiry shifts away from conflict that has arisen inevitably, as the result of the irreconcilable urges in human nature. Instead the analyst must think about the *conditions* under which conflict may (or may not) occur. This directs attention outward, into the patient's interpersonal reality. Fenichel's vision kept better faith with clinical work than Rapaport did, but he lost some of Freud's sense of the conflict inherent in life itself.

Drive aims precede experience; the drives are with us at birth and their nature is fixed phylogenetically. They cannot be dissected into simpler elements on the basis of psychological evidence. This is the core of Freud's rationalist perspective. But it cannot be sustained by the drive concept as it has been redefined by some of the theorists discussed here. In the terms of each revision there is significant interpersonal experience before there is drive. Not only that, but the particular characteristics of the drive itself are determined by the way that primitive needs were met in the earliest exchanges between infants and caretakers.

For Jacobson, although undifferentiated energy will bifurcate eventually, the process is inextricably linked to the experiences of infancy. For Schur and others who equate drive with wish, the perceptions and memories associated with needs are constituents of the drive itself. For Loewald and Kernberg, the drive is a motivational tendency that emerges from and is shaped by early object relations. Despite the differences in nuance, the implication of these formulations is the same: drive is not the irreducible and unconditioned force that ultimately creates experience.

Clinically, this leads to a whole range of questions that would tend not to arise within the terms of Freud's drive theory. The sexual or destructive impulse itself cannot be, despite Loewald's claim, "the most primitive unit of motivation." It must be dissected, despite Freud's claim that it could not be. An impulse—any impulse—acquires its particular characteristics over time, as a consequence of its history. There is no one place that a particular piece of analysis can stop, no interpretive bedrock on which everything else is built.

Drive is also a constitutional variable. Drive endowment, the strength and balance of the two drives, differs among different people. This characteristic of drive reflects the clinical effect of Freud's rationalist sensibility. It accounts for why behavior is so variable and why it is not simply mandated by environmental pressures. It also explains, to the drive theorist, why different people will have vastly different experiences even under similar stimulus conditions.

But in terms of several of the strategies discussed here, variations in experience depend on differences in the behavior of the object rather than on the subject's inner state. This shift in clinical sensibility dates back to Hartmann. When he suggested that perception is an autonomous ego function fueled by noninstinctual energy, he opened up the possibility that the "objects" of perception may be experienced unconditionally, independent of the influence of endogenous need (see Greenberg, 1986). This implication is developed more forcefully in the strategies that reject Freud's rationalism. Even the most conservative of these, the strategy of initial energic undifferentiation, assumes that the balance of instinctual forces itself will be largely determined by the relative strength of early good and bad relationships.

If the relationship shapes the drive, the importance of innate variation fades. Consider the way Loewald (1969) discusses some patients' intractable negative therapeutic reactions. Staying with the language of drive theory, Loewald suggests that these reactions result from unusually intense operations of the death instinct. But he does not attribute this to innate drive endowment, as Freud generally did. Instead Loewald believes that the intensity of the death instinct itself reflects an especially severe disturbance of preoedipal object relations.

The question for drive theorists from Freud on was always centered on the unique way that each of us constructs an experiential world. The theory correctly predicts that no two people can ever have the same expe-

rience. The differences that appeared were explained as the effect of innate variations in need, which decisively shaped perception. To take a commonplace example, harsh fathers were not necessarily hostile and competitive men; they were ordinary men seen through the lens of their sons' particularly intense incestuous or parricidal urges. Without theoretical support for some pre-experiential force behind individual difference, the focus shifts from what patients made of things to what happened to them. There is less thought about what the child wanted, and more awareness of the nature of the parent.

THE INTERPRETIVE system embodied in Freud's libido/aggression theory has enormous power to illuminate the hidden recesses of psychic life. It also has great limitations. The theory has been responsible for advances in the understanding of human accomplishments and afflictions, but it has also guided many analyses to a dead end. I have argued in this chapter that many Freudian theorists have defined away the dual-instinct theory. They have shed some of the narrow confines of the model, but they have also lost much that is compelling about it. They have lost its focus on the innate tendencies that give shape to our experience and make a life idiosyncratically our own. They have also lost a sensitivity to the inevitability of conflict that pervades every facet of life and gives psychoanalysis its tragic vision. Psychoanalysis, after all these theoretical revisions, is burdened with a theory of drive without meaning.

Drive in the Relational Model

W.R.D. FAIRBAIRN summarized the need to shift to an object relations psychology by quoting one patient's protest: "You're always talking about my wanting this and that desire satisfied; but what I really want is a father" (1946, p. 137). Fairbairn's use of the remark is clever, and his patient's plea is compelling (perhaps clever as well). It is appealing to think that what we really want is not crude indulgence—of desire or even of need— but a deeper relatedness. We should not, however, allow the poignance of what the patient said to mask its vagueness. As analysts we are obliged to ask a further question: "What, then, is a father?"

Once the question is raised, what had seemed obvious goes up in smoke. A father is a protector and an enemy, a companion and a rival, a lover and a murderer, a remote authority and the most intimate confidant. He can be, and generally is, all of these in the course of a single day, even at the same moment. There are infinite possible meanings to the experience of *Father,* vastly different for each of us. So what was Fairbairn's patient asking for? To know, we have to deepen our understanding of the particular configuration of being loved, bested, cared for, even hated, that he longed for in his plea. Nowhere is our task more literally *analytic;* we unravel the intricate tapestry of needs and desires that makes a man father to a particular patient.

The task, Freud insisted, cannot be accomplished from the outside. The desired father is less a figure in the external world than the embodiment of a pattern of satisfactions and disappointments, hopes and fears, passions and impressions, that runs through the patient's life. In his plea, the patient is trying to reconjure his own creation. It is a creation that can only be understood within the terms of its history, inextricably tied to the pa-

tient's passionate needs. For Freud there is no father without libido and aggression.

The vision invites excess. See where it led the French analyst Sascha Nacht: "the phenomena with which we are concerned must be considered by us on the level of needs and of functions resulting from the latter" (1952, p. 55). And what of everything else that contributes to our experience? There *was* a man around while Fairbairn's patient was growing up; didn't he have some effect on what the patient thinks a father is and on what he wants now? Not according to Nacht: "it is at best useless to burden the idea of reality with the diverse forms under which it may appear . . . it is sufficient—I should even say, preferable—to conceive of [reality] in the classic sense; i.e., as a principle. The rest concerns the sociologists" (p. 59).

In the last chapter I described a widespread convergence of opinion within "orthodox" psychoanalysis that need cannot adequately account for the intricacies of human motivation or experience. The consensus, I believe, goes further: the challenge to drive theory arises out of what analysts have learned about the significance and subtlety of social experience. The elaborated study of human relationships, most notably within the transference but outside it as well, has led many contemporary analysts to conclude that the dual-instinct theory has become a procrustean bed; the data no longer fit comfortably. Not only Freud's particular drive theory but the philosophical rationalism beneath any view of drive are subject to challenge.

Nacht saw what was coming. For many theorists, the conceptual slack caused by the weakening of the libido/aggression theory could be taken up by enlarging the psychodynamic role of reality. Loewenstein made it explicit. When they are better understood, he said, external factors will explain many of the phenomena that Freud understood in energic terms (1965, p. 49). What has evolved slowly (and partially) within Freudian circles has developed more forcefully outside them. Analysts operating within the relational model of the mind are united in their claim that it is misguided to begin theorizing with drive. Drive, these theorists believe, is *conceptually* misleading; the problem is not simply the specific qualities of libido and aggression. In the empiricist philosophical tradition, relational analysts look to what can be perceived around us: we should not emphasize endogenous determinants of experience; the qualities of relationships themselves are decisive.

The relational model contains many theories with different emphases

and nuances. But the hub from which the various perspectives radiate is the psychodynamic importance of social reality. Mitchell captures the central point that relational theorists want to make: "*what is inherent is not necessarily formative;* it does not push and shape experience, but is itself shaped by the relational context" (1988, p. 4). Thus, "Psychological meaning is . . . negotiated through interaction" (p. 5).

Drive, in the view of relational theorists, is not an unconditioned, irreducible, pre-experiential force that accounts for our deepest motives and generates its own experiential categories. There is no such force. Desires and needs derived from the drives do not bring people together, as Freud claimed they do (see especially Freud, 1921). Desires and needs do not exist in a psychologically meaningful way prior to a relationship. Even the most obviously endogenous elements in human functioning (Mitchell acknowledges temperament, bodily events, patterns of sensitivity and regulation, and so on) acquire their meaning through interpersonal negotiation. Sullivan (1953) recognized the "zonal needs" (those aimed at maintaining physiological homeostasis), saw that these were presocial and even pre-experiential, but dismissed them as characteristics of an animal, not a person. The person—and only the person is of interest to the psychiatrist, by Sullivan's definition—does not exist outside a social context.

My purpose in this chapter is to investigate an essential premise of the relational model: it is unnecessary and misleading to build theory around any concept of a pre-experiential force that brings people into relationships with others. Put another way, I will address the claims of relational theorists that they have created a drive-free psychoanalysis. I will try to show that they have not, in fact, done so. Their formulations mask an implicit drive theory that explains why the relationship exists in the first place, and what it means to each of the participants. I will use a case-study method, focusing on two important relational approaches: Fairbairn's "object relations theory" and Kohut's "psychology of the self." These models have led to a great deal of clinical and theoretical development. And both authors explicitly claim to have eliminated Freud's drives from their systems, making it necessary to ask what they have put in their conceptual place.

Once we look at the implicit drives in object relations theory and self psychology, we can more meaningfully compare these relational approaches with Freud's dual-instinct theory. To date these comparisons have not been quite fair: they have matched the libido/aggression theory against putatively drive-free theories. The limitations of the libido/aggres-

sion theory (especially its narrowness) have been widely documented, but questions have not been raised about similar constraints stemming from the "drive theories" of relational analysts.

Fairbairn's Object Relations Theory

Claiming that he was creating "an object relations theory of the personality," in 1952 Fairbairn announced a psychoanalytic model based on a radical confrontation with Freud's drive theory. Confusingly (but in a tradition of dissidents stretching from Jung to Kernberg), he retained the term "libido" while redefining it drastically. Libido, Fairbairn tells us repeatedly, is not pleasure-seeking. Rather, its aim is to bring people together with their objects. "The ultimate goal of libido is the object," he writes in a typical formulation (1941, p. 31). The significance of erotogenic zones is not that they provide the leading source of pleasure; they are a "sign-post" or "channel" to the object (1941, p. 33; 1946, p. 138).

Our natural human tendencies propel us toward the object, Fairbairn says, implying that we need say nothing more about what is innate. Once that basic premise is established, our attention is directed away from what motivated the relationship and toward its effects. Here is how he put it:

> it is high time that psychopathological inquiry, which in the past has been successively focused, first upon impulse, and later upon the ego, should now be focused upon *the object* towards which impulse is directed. To put the matter more accurately if less pointedly, the time is now ripe for a psychology of *object-relationships* . . . From the point of view which I have now come to adopt, psychology may be said to resolve itself into a study of the relationships of the individual to his objects (1946, p. 60).

Fairbairn's intention, then, is to create a drive-free psychoanalysis, a theory that can begin with the relationship itself. How successful has he been?

Stephen Mitchell believes that Fairbairn achieved what he set out to do. Accordingly, in reading Fairbairn he goes along with the expressed intention and begins with the idea that the child approaches objects seeking "contact, emotional exchange." But people are complex and relationships are difficult, so an intricate drama unfolds:

> The parents' capacity to be reached and moved by the child is necessarily obscured by and hostage to the vulnerabilities and conflicts of the character structure of the individual parent. Human beings are deceptively elusive creatures, which makes object seeking, the search for access to and connection

with others an engrossing and intricate process . . . the object seeking Fairbairn speaks of is a very complex, subtle process. Each parent is accessible in some situations, inaccessible in others; in some ways reachable, in some ways always out of reach. If *object seeking is to be regarded as a fundamental human motivation,* we are referring . . . to a complex array of desires, identifications, and behaviors which reflect efforts to reach others (1988, pp. 104–105, my italics).

With this, Mitchell has given us a compelling rendering of Fairbairn, and from this he creatively synthesizes his version of Fairbairn with the sensibilities of other relational theorists. He goes on to develop a vision of behavior and experience that has been formed (and deformed) by the particular blend of parental strength, vulnerability, elusiveness, and accessibility that characterized early relations.

But Fairbairn begged an important question, and Mitchell lets him get away with it. The question is this: What does the child seek in seeking that object? What is the *nature* of the contact, or of the emotional exchange, that the child wants with the parents? Certainly it is not *any* contact, because many varieties of exchange between people are patently aversive to all concerned.

Eventually, as Fairbairn argues persuasively, people come to prefer relationships with bad objects to having no object relationships at all. They even prefer familiar bad objects to new objects that potentially offer better qualities of relatedness (Fairbairn, 1943, 1958). But this only implies that there is something inherently good about the feeling of familiarity; it hardly addresses the problem of why somebody would seek a bad relationship in the first place.

Before the bad relationship gets established as a familiar psychic presence, there must be certain characteristics of the exchange that the child is moved to seek. Freud was clear (if narrow and probably incorrect) about what these are: the kinds of exchange that satisfy our biologically determined needs and lead to pleasurable sensations. The needs, in turn, are those specified by the libido/aggression theory.

What determines the needs that Fairbairn has in mind? Mitchell says that the child's desires are complex, but while that captures the experience of the analyst trying to make sense of what patients want, it is not a good enough answer to a theoretical question. Psychoanalysis requires an interpretive system, and this demands a commitment to finding some order within the complexity of human motivation.

Although it has been masked by the more radical idea that libido is

object-seeking, Fairbairn's is a theory that begins, as Freud's did, with biology and that works the same way conceptually.* In my view, Fairbairn's drive theory is based on a rather simple notion of what the child wants: it is a one-drive model based on self-preservative needs manifested in the child's (and later in the adult's) dependency.

If I can make a case for this reading of Fairbairn, it will be no more correct to say that he saw object seeking as a fundamental human motive than to say that Freud did. Freud's sexual and aggressive drives require an object in the same way that Fairbairn's dependency needs do. The difference is not in the object seeking; it lies in the nature of the hypothesized need.†

Early on, Fairbairn took a position that he never abandoned:

> The first social relationship established by the individual is that between himself and his mother; and the focus of this relationship is the suckling situation, in which his mother's breast provides the focal point of his libidinal object, and his mouth the focal point of his own libidinal attitude (1940, pp. 10–11).

Although it seems like a conventional version of things, importing the theory of libidinal development proposed by Freud and Abraham, we still have to ask how Fairbairn gets the impression that "the focus of this relationship is the suckling situation." Why does he believe that the mouth is "most important of all, the first means of intimate social contact" (p. 10)?

Perhaps Fairbairn would say that he is simply passing on his observations of the events of infancy. But what he has told us is neither an observation nor is it simple; it is a theoretical statement that collapses the data of observation into a specific conceptual category. Certainly there are other observable dimensions of the infant's relationship to its mother. There are visual, auditory, tactile, and affective exchanges. There is mutuality, the reciprocity that has been frequently described in the literature of psychoanalytically informed developmental research (Stern, 1985; Beebe and Lachmann, 1988a,b; Lichtenberg, 1983a). It takes neither a psychoana-

---

*I don't mean by this that Fairbairn's drive operates according to the pleasure or the constancy principles, as Freud's drives do. In any case, the regulatory principles are not intrinsic to the drive concept; they address the problem of how the mind handles stimuli. Here I am referring to the conceptual role of drive in the theoretical structure that each author has developed.

†It is true that in Fairbairn's theory the object is necessarily human, while in Freud's it is not (and may of course be autoerotic). But Fairbairn claims a more radical departure.

lyst nor a developmental researcher to notice these things; all it takes is watching infants and their caretakers.

I have no doubt that Fairbairn was aware of how rich the qualities of relatedness are from the very beginnings of life. And yet he centered all of them on orality. How did he decide which is the theme and which are its variations? The decision depends on a crucial assumption: "the oral incorporative tendency is the most fundamental of all tendencies" (1940, p. 14). But if that is true, consider what orality is: it is a "fundamental tendency" that generates and organizes a range of object-related experiences. This makes it look very much like the Rosetta Stone that the drives were for Freud (Ogden, 1984).

As Fairbairn developed his formulation, further similarities to Freud's drives emerged. Orality, he says, determines the nature of the child's experience of both self and object. Thus the infant's ego is a "mouth ego" (1940, p. 10), and the first "natural and biological" object is the breast (1941, p. 31). He criticized Abraham's history of the emergence of libidinal phases, insisting that while the breast and the genitals are natural objects, others (especially feces) are not. This distinction can only be based on some underlying motivational theory. Otherwise what does it mean to say that an object is "natural"? The breast and the genitals are natural objects because they are well suited to satisfy certain biologically determined needs. Fairbairn characterized orality as a fundamental tendency because it is the earliest expression of what is, for all intents and purposes, the child's self-preservative drive.

The importance of the mother as a person and as a "natural object" follows (much as it did for Freud) from her ability to meet the child's drive-derived needs. Mother is of interest to the child because she has a breast. Thus, "when the biological history of early childhood is considered, it becomes plain that there is only one natural part-object, viz. the breast of the mother, and that the most significant whole object is the mother—with the father as rather a poor second" (1941, p. 40). This sensibility cannot be supported by an object-seeking drive. If all the child wanted was an object, why would he seek mother in preference to father? The preference for mother is predetermined in Fairbairn's system; it is not dictated by the psychodynamic configurations within the family or by any other interpersonal reality. Fairbairn is not talking about one parent being more *available* than another; he is talking about one parent being more *suitable* as a drive object. The child prefers his mother because self-preservation drives him toward her.

Even psychological dependence is secondary to self-preservation in Fairbairn's system. Although the "greatest need of a child" is assurance that he is genuinely loved as a person and that his love is accepted (1941), this is neither the beginning nor the end of the story. The child needs assurance only because his "very helplessness . . . is sufficient to render him dependent in an unconditional sense" (1941, p. 47). Thus: "It is only in so far as such assurance is forthcoming in a form sufficiently convincing to enable him to depend safely upon his real objects that he is able gradually to renounce infantile dependence without misgiving" (p. 39). Evidently love—and the maintenance of the relationship itself—safeguards dependency needs. These dependency needs continue to haunt us throughout the course of life: "all psychopathological developments are ultimately based upon an infantile attitude of dependence" (1943, pp. 79–80n).

For Fairbairn, human nature is passive at its core. This is an essential implication of the way he formulated the self-preservative drive. The infant needs and wants only to be taken care of; there is nothing in Fairbairn's system to support a vision of the child (or even the adult) actively pursuing her own aims. This stands in stark contrast to Freud's drive theory, which is based on the assumption that drive aims are, by definition, actively pursued (1915a). The person is active even when the aims themselves require passive enactments.

If Freud's drive theory reveals the activity that lies behind apparently passive behavior, Fairbairn's theory suggests that apparent activity compensates for thwarted passivity. Consider his discussion of the infant's thumb sucking:

> Why does a baby suck his thumb? . . . If we answer that the baby sucks his thumb because his mouth is an erotogenic zone and sucking provides him with erotic pleasure, it may sound convincing enough; but we are really missing the point. To bring out the point, we must ask ourselves the further question—"Why his thumb?" And the answer to this question is—"Because there is no breast to suck." Even the baby must have a libidinal object; and, if he is deprived of his natural object (the breast), he is driven to provide an object for himself. Thumb-sucking thus represents a technique for dealing with an unsatisfactory object-relationship (1941, p. 33).

Two of Fairbairn's central hypotheses lie behind this piece of analysis. First, apparently erotic activities are more deeply understood as ways of establishing and maintaining object relationships. Second, the recourse to autoerotism becomes necessary because the natural relationship has failed.

Because there is "no breast to suck," the infant is driven to a compensatory exercise in self-stimulation and gratification. If there were a breast to suck, the infant would suck it.

There are several things wrong with this analysis. Perhaps most obviously (and in a sense, most trivially) it fails on empirical grounds. Fairbairn could not have anticipated the advent of *in utero* photography, but we know now that the fetus sucks its thumb in the womb, as early as the fourth or fifth month after conception (Rugh and Shettles, 1971; Nilsson, 1990). Virtually by definition (certainly by Fairbairn's definition) there could have been no failed object relationship by that time; in any case, there surely was no lost breast. *In utero* sucking cannot be provoked by object loss.

More important, Fairbairn's way of looking at things gives thumb sucking a bad name, because it is shaped by his conviction about the child's passivity. Consider the image of the thumb-sucker that emerges from his description. It begins with the infant in a dependent relationship with an unavailable object. Everything that Fairbairn understands about what happens next, everything he says about what the infant does, hinges on his having begun the analysis at this point. Because the infant has been abandoned and deprived, it is driven to autoerotism and to establishing relations with internal objects, which are pathological by definition (1941, p. 34). The only reason for an infant to suck its thumb is to compensate for a failed relationship.

Consider what Fairbairn does not notice, or what he sees but discounts: the pleasure the infant feels in sucking its thumb; the experience of agency involved in doing something for itself; the effects of both the pleasure and the sense of agency on feelings about itself as a developing person. None of this matters, since it is all subordinated to the impact of the absent breast. Pleasure seeking may be a narrow way of understanding the motive behind thumb sucking, but it does emphasize the infant's active strivings. Fairbairn's theoretical commitment led him to overlook these active tendencies.

Certainly some children will suck their thumbs when the object is absent, and it is important to address their experience of loss and the compensatory aspects of their behavior. But there are other perspectives to consider. Because Fairbairn is so focused on the child's need to be cared for, he can see only what the child has lost; he misses the child's interest in and evolving capacity to care for itself—including providing pleasure for itself. Thumb sucking, and other autoerotic activities, contribute to

building a sense of competence. This in turn provides the background for the child's private, self-contained enjoyment of itself, its body, and its capacity to create pleasurable sensations *autonomously*. This will eventually provide a way of coping with the absence of the object, but it will also be the basis of many characteristics of healthy maturity—those having to do with the derivatives of pleasure-seeking trends (creativity, productivity, and such). Thumb sucking—whatever motivates it—is a route to autonomy and individuation; it is not simply the beginning of pathological relationships with internal objects.

The Psychology of the Self

The structure of self psychology is similar to that of Fairbairn's object relations theory in one crucial respect: a need *for* a relationship moves the individual *toward* the relationship. Once that has happened, our attention—clinically and theoretically—is directed toward the relationship itself. "The primary units," Kohut wrote, "are *ab initio* the complex experiences and action patterns of a self/self-object unit" (1977, p. 249). As analysts, we begin with the relationship; from this starting point we will be concerned with its effects on the person's developmental history or psychopathology.

Because of this shift in emphasis, the psychodynamic importance of endogenous motivational forces wanes, and the slack is taken up by the vicissitudes of exchanges between child and caretakers. Behaviors once explained as the workings of unmodulated, innately determined impulse (perverse sexuality, raw aggression, unrestrained oral greed) are reinterpreted as the inevitable consequences of failed relatedness. Kohut, like Fairbairn, is adamant that he has rejected drive theory. What had once been understood as driven behavior becomes a "disintegration product" reflecting the effects of this failure. Eventually drive itself succumbs to the shift in perspective: Kohut dismissed it as "a vague and insipid biological concept" (1982, p. 401). He put his reformulation of the interpretive system of psychoanalysis this way: "it is not a libidinal drive that, psychologically speaking, attains its momentum in the child, but . . . from the beginning, the drive experience is subordinated to the child's experience of the relation between the self and the self-objects" (1977, p. 80).

Just what this changed sensibility means interpretively pivots on the notion of a "selfobject." Kohut thought so himself: he characterized the selfobject as the "crucial theoretical concept" of his new framework (1977,

p. xiii). The idea of a *self*object distinguishes self psychology from other relational theories. Had Kohut simply said that the importance of drive is subordinated to the child's experience of the relations between herself and her objects, he would have added nothing to what had already been said by Winnicott, Fairbairn, and Sullivan. But he is saying something more, something about the kind of relationship that makes a person a selfobject.

If I can ask, as I did at the beginning of this chapter, what a father is, I can certainly ask what a selfobject is. What does someone do to become the selfobject of another person? Why does someone become a selfobject instead of becoming a different kind of object, or simply remaining an indifferent "other"? Kohut and his followers suggest that a person becomes a selfobject because he or she offers a particular *quality* of relatedness. To put it another way, a selfobject is a person who does certain sorts of things for another, and just what these things are is determined by the person's needs. A selfobject, then, is a person who responds in a particular way to specifiable, pre-experiential needs. Without the needs, there could be no selfobject—the needs give shape to the experience and endow the relationship with its special meaning.

This sounds very similar to the way in which a thing (human or not, animate or not) becomes an object in Freud's drive theory. An object is a thing that has become the target or a drive, and it has been targeted because it is suited to satisfy a need or because historically it has satisfied some need. "Repeated situations of satisfaction," Freud wrote, "have created an object out of the mother" (1926, p. 170). The kind of object that *mother* is (a breast, a rival, a lover) depends on the nature of the need, and that in turn is specified by the drive theory.

Despite the efforts of self psychologists to distance themselves from this type of formulation, the route to becoming a selfobject is remarkably like what Freud described. Howard Bacal has recently offered a revealing example:

> a gasoline station attendant whose inability to provide fuel because the pumps are empty has no effect on the customer's sense of self at some moment, and the customer will simply shrug his shoulders and drive on to another gas station. At another moment, of course, when his self-state renders him vulnerable to selfobject failure, the customer might experience the gas station attendant as having a significant effect on his sense of self, and react quite strongly (1990, p. 206).

With this, Bacal asserts that the nature of the driver's experience of the attendant, the kind of object the attendant is for the driver, is fully ex-

plained by the changes in some underlying need. The attendant will become a selfobject if (and only if) the driver's needs reach a certain threshold of intensity.

This formulation is compatible, if not identical, with the sensibility of Freud's drive theory. The libido theory predicts that intensified sexual need (for example, the analysand's growing sexual tension following the analyst's enforcement of the rule of abstinence) will create an object out of someone who otherwise was not: thus, transference. Bacal's example is striking because, like Freud, he says nothing about any transactional determinants of whether the attendant actually becomes a selfobject. Selfobject theory shares more of Freud's philosophical rationalism than meets the eye at first. Nothing that the other person *does* seems to matter. The behavior or attitude of the other is irrelevant; the nature of the relationship and the person's experience of the object are defined entirely by the need.

Because of this, it is reasonable to suggest that the concept of a selfobject has a *motivational* theory—even a drive theory—built into it. Basch, in fact, goes so far as to suggest that self psychology "replaces the dual instinct theory of motivation with the selfobject theory of motivation" (1987, p. 375). We could continue the parallel with Fairbairn and say that people are moved to seek selfobjects. But this would beg the same key question that Fairbairn begged: the why (and even the what) of object seeking. We again encounter the problem: What are the "drives" of self psychology?

The question is best answered by considering the history of Kohut's theoretical revisionism. Like Fairbairn, Kohut began by retaining the term "libido" while redefining it. But his initial step was more conservative. In maintaining that libido was object-seeking rather than pleasure-seeking, Fairbairn was trying to change the theory at its core. Kohut, in contrast, added a new kind of libido to the system. Narcissistic libido, an independent energy with its own developmental course, reflects a previously unidentified but equally innate need of the child's. Accordingly, the object of narcissistic libido is in certain respects more like the object of Freud's theory than like the object of Fairbairn's. Fairbairn's object is a fact of life; without it, we could not even talk meaningfully of an ego. In contrast, the selfobject is important—even necessary in the sense that food and oxygen are important and necessary. But the object is not, strictly speaking, there from the beginning. Instead it *becomes* important, and it does so because it serves the child's developmental need. In Kohut's original formulation, the need is for the development of two poles of the self. One of these poles

is organized around the child's belief in his own perfection, expressed by a natural and healthy exhibitionism; the other is based in the experience of merger with an idealized other (Kohut, 1971). These needs and the relationships to which they give rise are very different from those determined by object libido, as Freud described them and as Kohut made them a part of his own system. But the process of object formation is similar, regardless of which "libidinal" needs the object serves.

With the advent of the psychology of the self in the broader sense (Kohut, 1977) and in the development of Kohut's theory by his followers, the idea of narcissistic libido has all but disappeared. Bacal writes: "In self psychological theory, instinctual motivation is explicitly rejected as a factor of psychological significance" (1990, p. 198). This leaves the theory with no fully articulated, independent concept of the inner need that leads the person to others and makes another person into a selfobject. The theory at that point is similar to Fairbairn's: what Basch called the "selfobject theory of motivation" has the same tone as Fairbairn's claim that he has created an "object relations theory of the personality."

Kohut's ideas about narcissistic libido continue to influence the way the concept of a selfobject is understood. Definitions focus on those qualities in a relationship that advance the cause of self-cohesion.* Ornstein says that the selfobject is "related to only in terms of the specific, phase-appropriate needs of the developing self" (1978, p. 60). Stolorow and Lachmann express a similar point of view when they say that the selfobject is one which "serves to restore or maintain the sense of self" (1980, p. 1n; see also similar definitions in Wolf, 1985; Bacal, 1990).

The definition is not particularly useful. It fails us clinically just where we need the help of theory, because it does not address the critical question of what happens between two people to "restore or maintain the sense of self" of one of them. Exchanges between people affect the sense of self of both participants; nobody could work long as an analyst without noticing

---

*Because of this, there is one line of thought in the definition of a selfobject that has to do with its differentiation from the self. At the outset, this was central to the definition: selfobjects were thought to be experienced as part of the self and as operating within the subject's orbit of control (Kohut, 1971). There is no longer agreement on the point. Ornstein (1978) and Stolorow and Lachmann (1980) include it in their definitions. Goldberg (1988) implies that it is not essential, and Bacal (1990) is explicit that selfobjects may be experienced as external to the self. Wolf suggests a third possibility: that selfobjects are experienced simultaneously as within and outside the self (1983, p. 314). There is enough disagreement on the point that the "location" of selfobjects can no longer be considered one of the concept's defining characteristics.

that. Many different theoretical systems include some ideas about what aspects of the relationship are most important in this respect. Analysts who rely on the dual-instinct theory, for example, say that the object's response to a person's vital needs (sexual and aggressive by definition) are the most important determinants of the sense of self. This implication of the drive theory was an especially important part of Winnicott's and Jacobson's way of using it to understand both development and clinical process. If an object's reaction to drive-determined needs enhances the sense of self, it is experienced as a good object; if not, it is a bad object.

These definitions of selfobject fail, therefore, to differentiate a selfobject from what would be considered a good object in any psychoanalytic theory. Bacal is not stretching things when he says that "bad objects would be those who fail to fulfill a selfobject function when they are expected to do so" (1990, p. 216). The opposite of selfobject is bad object.

Is there something that differentiates a selfobject from a traditional "good object"? If not, we would have to consider the possibility that self psychology is simply a restatement of traditional psychoanalysis with its deepest explanatory principles excised. But there is more to it than that. I would suggest this: the difference lies in the kinds of needs that are presumed to affect the sense of self. To put it another way, the difference is in the kinds of drives that determine human behavior and experience.

What are these drives? This can be a difficult question to answer because self psychologists most of the time tend to talk about the irreducible "needs of the self"—self-cohesion, self-actualization, self-regulation, and so on. This reflects Kohut's insistence that theorizing on the molar, presumably experience-near level of self is more psychoanalytic than talking on the molecular, presumably experience-distant level of need (1977, pp. 69–83).

I suggest, however, that we can get beyond this theoretical posturing and find an answer to our question by looking at the way different self psychologists specify selfobject *functions*. Functions make a person into a selfobject. Bacal's gas station attendant would have been a selfobject if he had given the driver gas; he was a bad object because he did not. It is the selfobject's functions that have an impact on the person's sense of self. It is fair to say that "selfobject function" is simply another way of saying "the needs of the self."

When he first introduced the concept of the selfobject, Kohut specified two principal functions. First there is mirroring: the child displays his developing capacities to the selfobject, who admires them with a gleam in

his eye. This encourages a healthy grandiosity and exhibitionism, characteristics that will facilitate the child's ability to pursue future ambitions in a joyous, effective way. Later the selfobject must also permit idealization, in which he is admired for his own perfection, allowing the child to merge with the omnipotence he sees in the other. This permits the development of ideals and values that can act as guiding principles throughout life.

Both Kohut and his followers quickly decided that these two selfobject functions were too limiting. Shortly after he introduced psychology of the self in the broader sense, Kohut (1980) suggested that more selfobject functions should be enumerated. Many different self psychologists have attempted to do so. The result is considerable disagreement about both the number and the nature of selfobject functions. The situation is parallel to the disagreement about the number and quality of drives encountered among classical analysts.

Despite his idea that more should be said about the qualities of selfobject relations, Kohut did not do so himself. In his own writings, mirroring and idealization remained the superordinate selfobject functions. He translated these functions into needs of the self this way: "the need of the budding self for the joyful response of the mirroring selfobject, the need of the budding self for the omnipotent selfobject's pleased acceptance of its merger needs, are primary configurations" (1975, p. 788). Essentially, the functions of mirroring and permitting idealization are phase-specific means by which the selfobject meets the child's need for acceptance (see Friedman, 1980). Like Fairbairn, Kohut arrived at a one-drive theory. His followers who remain content with generalizing about the selfobject contributing positively to the sense of self are also left with a one-drive model (for example, Ornstein, 1978).

When Kohut's followers picked up the suggestion that more selfobject functions could be named, the number of "primary configurations" or fundamental needs ramified. Bacal (1990) illustrates the potential range. In his list of selfobject functions he includes: satisfying libidinal and aggressive drives; regulating tension and affect; providing an experience of safety, recognition, and support; and providing meaning to internal and external experience. Bacal does not intend his list to be complete, although he does believe that the various functions reflect independent needs that cannot be derived from more fundamental needs. He has built on Kohut's framework to create the self-psychological counterpart of a multiple-drive model.

As a final indication of how the concept of selfobject function can be

expanded to include whatever needs an author feels are most fundamental, consider Ernest Wolf's discussion of the developmental line of selfobject relations (1980). At the beginning of life, Wolf writes, "the primary need is for selfobject relations that lend organization to the emerging self." These needs are met by the mirroring and idealizing relationships with selfobjects that Kohut described. But when things go well, some self-consolidation is achieved and the need shifts. The quality of the relationship with selfobjects changes accordingly. Wolf then speaks of "confronting the selfobject as an antagonist against whom self-assertion mobilizes healthy aggression that promotes the cohesive strength of the self" (pp. 125, 126).

Consistent with the terms of self psychology, Wolf conceptualizes this shift as a change in the nature of the needed relationship with the selfobject, a change that requires the selfobject to behave in a different way. An "antagonist" selfobject can hardly act like the accepting figure that Kohut envisioned. But, beyond that, he has departed considerably from Kohut's theory of the nature of fundamental human needs. Where Kohut had talked of healthy assertiveness that decompensates into aggression as the result of selfobject failure (1977, p. 116), Wolf believes that there is an original, irreducible, healthy aggression, presumably independent of thwarted assertiveness. Wolf approaches the task of theoretical revision by proposing a new selfobject function, but his deeper purpose is to suggest a new and profoundly different vision (within self psychology) of the relationship between aggressive and assertive needs (see also Lachmann, 1986).

THE CONCEPT of selfobject function, like the concept of drive, is fluid enough to permit specification in a variety of ways. Within the broad spectrum of self psychology there are many visions of what motivates human relationships. When Freud thought about his drive theory, he often wondered how many and what sorts of drives there were (for example, 1915a, p. 124). The same questions could be asked about selfobject functions. But the idea of a selfobject is not simply motivational; it adds something beyond what drive connotes conceptually. Consider what is implied when self psychologists speak of a selfobject "function." Referring to a function directs attention away from the need of the subject and toward the behavior of the object. The person who is the object of a drive (if indeed the object is a person, or even sensate) is a more or less accidental participant in the child's internal drama; he may well be oblivious of his status as an

object. This is often the case when movie stars, sports figures, or other famous people become the objects of their admirers. They are objects in the fullest sense of the term, although they have no way of knowing it. In contrast, the sensibility of self psychology suggests that the child's needs constitute a claim on the selfobject; they impose an obligation. Normal development requires that these needs be met—in contrast to the needs of the dual-instinct theory, which never can be fully met, even in principle.

We can express the difference between Freud's drives and the functions of the selfobject in this way: while drive determines the subject's *experience* of the object, selfobject functions determine the object's *responsibility* to the subject. In this sense, the needs that give rise to selfobject functions are like those that determine Mahler's phases of separation/individuation. The child's need to experience a symbiotic merger, then to separate and individuate, like the needs of the self that Kohut describes, prescribe an optimal response. The parent (especially the mother) must act in a certain way if development is to proceed normally.

As self psychologists enumerate more and more functions, the sense of the selfobject's fiduciary responsibility to the child remains constant. Thoughts about "optimal" or "proper" or "appropriate" responses color discussions of the relationship. As a result, the more functions added to the system, the more complicated life becomes for the selfobject.

This sensibility has an important effect on how self psychologists understand the clinical process. Consider Bacal's discussion of negative transference and resistance:

> In my experience, when the selfobject relationship with the analyst is in place as a stable "background," conflicts and deficits . . . in relation to others will variously occupy the foreground, and those which emerge in relation to the analyst will not be experienced as unduly problematic. When the selfobject relationship between the patient and his analyst becomes disturbed, however, conflicts and deficits in relation to him will occupy center stage. It is at this juncture that "resistance" becomes a consideration (1990, pp. 210–211).

This sounds a bit like Freud in *Studies on Hysteria*. Transference and resistance are not central features of the analytic process—they are disruptions. Related and more important is the implication that any disruption in the smooth flow of therapeutic progress is traceable to something in the analyst's reactions, understanding, or character. Negative or aversive reactions do not have a life of their own; they do not reflect (or serve) any kind of internal process. Instead, they are always reactive; their occurrence is evi-

dence of some failure of the analyst's. The analyst, like other selfobjects, is obliged by the patient's "needs."

Is a Drive-Free Theory Possible?

Despite their attempts Fairbairn, Kohut, and Kohut's followers within self psychology have not been able to create a drive-free theoretical system. They have not dispensed with drives entirely but have developed systems that begin with different drives, drives that replace Freud's. Is it simply that these theorists have failed to accomplish what they set out to do, or is the goal itself beyond reach? Is it possible to dispose of the dual-instinct theory without putting *something* in its conceptual place?

The philosopher Ortega y Gassett was fighting his own intellectual battles when he expressed what could be a manifesto for the relational model: "*Man has no nature; what he has is . . . history.* Expressed differently: what nature is to things, history . . . is to man" (1941, p. 217). Nature, as Ortega uses the term, is fixed and static. History seems much more alive, vital, human. If what we have to work with is history, we can begin with what Mitchell describes as meaning negotiated through interaction. History means that our subject is the person in action, inextricably woven into a social tapestry.

On this view, the endogenous determinants of experience (which Ortega would call nature) are inconsequential. Theory begins with the relationship itself. This is where Fairbairn and Kohut, each in his own way, claimed to begin. But, at the risk of perseveration, let me ask: What *is* the relationship? What do we look at, even when all we are after is a simple description? Schafer has identified the problem in literary terms: "The allegedly factual world provides a plenitude of facts to speak of, and what the analysand selects from this plenitude and the narrative versions of these facts that the analysand constructs are not inevitable" (1985, p. 539).

What is true of analysands applies equally to analysts. "The relationship" is too complex a phenomenon even to be described meaningfully. Before anything interesting can be said about it, it must be given a shape by the theorist. History textbooks don't read much like contemporary newspapers, and newspapers in turn don't record events as they were experienced by the participants. The differences lie in the principles that order the various narrative constructions. History is created when a theme is imposed on events.

That was precisely the purpose of Freud's drive theory. Giving shape to a relationship, he assumed, requires us to specify the forces that brought the participants together in the first place. We must also have in mind some vision of what continues to hold the participants together in a particular relationship. Without this we cannot understand what is happening. Consider the various ways a simple conversation can look to people who approach it with strong preconceptions. The drawn-out double entendre is a classic comic device in the theater. The joke depends on there being two very different sets of assumptions about what is going on. This is equally true, if less striking, in everyday life. *We cannot grasp meaning without some idea of motive.*

When we observe relationships psychoanalytically, our interpretation of what is going on is powerfully influenced by our theories about what people need from each other. Consider what may be the simplest example of this. Every psychoanalytic theory includes some idea that, from the beginning of life, the infant experiences relationships as either "good" or "bad." There are good and bad breasts (Klein), good and bad "me's" (Sullivan), good and bad objects (Fairbairn). The list could go on. But what makes a relationship good or bad? Is it that a need (hunger, for example) was satisfied? Is it something in the attitude of one participant toward the other? Do the feelings of both participants play a role? Is it that the feelings of one of the participants were or were not pleasant? And what is a "pleasant" feeling anyway? Trapped by his theoretical commitment to the constancy principle, Freud believed for many years in the unlikely assumption that stimulation is invariably unpleasant. Where, then, do we look in the complexity of even the simplest exchange to locate and define the goodness or badness that the infant is presumed to experience?

There is, I suggest, nothing good or bad about a relationship that is independent of what the participants want or need from it. Any theorist who characterizes a relationship as good or bad has some notion of the child's motives for being in the relationship in the first place. He may see the child as seeking pleasure or security or affirmation or stimulation; there are a great many possibilities. But always he has, within the terms I have described, a drive theory. It is important in this connection to point out that "contact" or "object seeking" or "attachment" cannot operate as a drive in this sense. None of these would allow a theorist to say that an observed relationship—one in which there is contact with an object—is nonetheless aversive or bad for the child. The judgment supposes that the child wants or needs something beyond the mere presence of the object.

For Freud and those who accepted the libido/aggression model, the relationship is good if it satisfies the most urgent of a variety of bodily based, maturationally changing sensual needs, evoking pleasurable feelings in the child. That is why Hartmann could comfortably assert this apparent contradiction: "so-called 'good' object relations may become a developmental handicap" (1952, p. 163). The kinds of satisfactions that make the child's experience of a relationship good are not necessarily the kinds that promote optimal ego development. This formulation would be incoherent for Kohut, who considered a relationship good and only if it fosters optimal development of the self. There are other ways of approaching the problem. Sullivan, in contrast to both Hartmann and Kohut, defined the earliest relationship—the relationship to the nipple—as good if it resulted in satisfaction of zonal needs and, perhaps most important, if it was uncontaminated by the mother's anxiety.

In each case, even gross assessment of the quality of the relationship depends on some theory of what the subject (the child in my examples) wants or needs from it. It is plausible that analysts operating from different models might arrive at very different judgments about whether a particular relationship is good or bad. And, since all analysts make that kind of judgment about their patients' experience, all analysts are working, at least implicitly, with some theory of unfolding developmental need.

Assumptions about need have implications beyond what an analyst thinks will be experienced as good or bad. They are important determinants of her understanding of the overall course of development. Just as every theory makes some judgment about good and bad experience, every theory has some concept of developmental phases or stages. The concept of a developmental phase hinges on presumed changes in the nature of need. In turn, it is assumed that the relative importance of different needs at different phases determines the quality of experience generally, and the experience of object relations in particular. When Freud, or Fairbairn, says that the child first experiences mother as a breast, it is because of what they assume the child needs or wants most. The sequence of libidinal phases in Freud's work extends this understanding over the entire course of childhood.

A different drive theory would imply an alternative sequence of developmental experience. Kohut, for example, never speaks of mothers as "breasts": at the earliest stage of life they are "mirroring selfobjects" because that is—in Kohut's view—what the child needs and is looking for in another person. Later they are idealized selfobjects (and later yet, in

Wolf's view, antagonists) because the nature of the need has changed. Mahler's description of the symbiotic mother and the mother of separation reflects her own assumptions about developmental need. I don't think it would ever have occurred to anybody to characterize a mother as a breast (and certainly not as a mirror) if they hadn't looked at the relationship between mother and child through the lens of some motivational assumption. A naive observer would notice that infants eat and that it seems important to them, but that is not all they do. Without a drive theory it would make as much sense to describe mother as a lap, a face, a temptress, or a soother.

Some lenses produce especially dramatic visions. Without his one-drive theory emphasizing dependency needs, Fairbairn could not have arrived at the idea that for the child a father is "chiefly . . . a parent without breasts" (1951, p. 174; also 1944, p. 122).

An equally impressive example of the way that a motivational theory influences the understanding of developmental experience appears in Fairbairn's formulation of the Oedipus complex. Again because he sees only dependency, he compresses the entire Oedipus complex into that theme:

> the deeper significance of the situation would appear to reside in the fact that it represents a differentiation of the single object of the ambivalent (later oral) phase into two objects, one being an accepted object, identified with one of the parents, and the other being a rejected object, identified with the remaining parent (1941, p. 37).

With this Fairbairn has collapsed the richness of the oedipal period—with its range of new wishes, feelings, and capacities—into a replay of the themes of earliest infancy. Because he is so monotonically focused on dependency, he is unable to notice that the child has *changed* during the first three or four years of life. The child approaches the parent at age three or four in a very different way than he did as an infant. Equally important, the parent approaches and reacts to the child differently. Fairbairn's understanding of the Oedipus complex provides an excellent example of what happens when an analyst is seduced by his theory.

Since motivation orders our judgment of relationships and our way of conceptualizing sequence, it is an inescapable element of psychoanalytic theory. Fairbairn and Kohut did not simply fail to execute their intention of creating a drive-free theory; their intention was unattainable from the beginning. Whether theorists are explicit about it or not, they are always working with some pre-experiential tendency that gives shape to relational

experience. Relational theorists differ from Freud in the sorts of drives they have substituted for libido and aggression, and in their failure to specify the nature of these drives.

Conflict in the Relational Model

Relational theories are especially weak in their conceptualization of conflict. This is most evident in Fairbairn's one-drive model and in the similar vision contained within Kohut's psychology of the self. In each framework, innate needs are unitary. Given an appropriately "good" or "facilitating" or "empathic" environment, these needs will be met, leading to feelings of satisfaction, to a sense of the goodness and competence of the self, and to convictions about the benevolence of the object world.

This is reflected in the kind of "self" envisioned by one-drive theorists. Fairbairn's unitary ego, Kohut's nascent self, and Winnicott's "true self" as well are poised to grow and to flourish. They will do so unless they are assailed by rejections (Fairbairn), failures (Kohut), or impingements (Winnicott). Conflict does not reflect the pressures of trying to satisfy essential but inescapably incompatible needs. It is not something inherent in the human condition. Instead, conflict arises from attempts to cope with the failure of others to respond adequately to needs that could (if the other were more available or more loving or less disturbed) be met, at least in principle.

Consider Fairbairn's thoughts on repression. He laments Freud's decision to base his theory on what Melanie Klein later called the depressive position rather than on the schizoid position (1951, pp. 168–169). This is a technical way of stating an important shift in clinical sensibility. As Fairbairn notes, Freud believed that repression is necessary because different thoughts (urges, wishes, memories, whatever) evoke intolerably ambivalent feelings. Klein's depressive position refers specifically to love and hate directed toward the same person, but Freud's original vision was broader: repression might be directed toward conflicting loyalties, incompatible wishes, intense fears, and so on (see Chapter 6). For Freud, repression is a way of coping with conflicting internal states.

In contrast, Fairbairn introduced the schizoid position to reflect what happens to the child when her objects cannot accept the child's love. The child's feelings at the very beginning are unitary and unambivalent. The problem lies entirely in the object's response, so that: "It is the great tragedy of the schizoid individual that his love seems to destroy; and it is

because his love seems so destructive that he experiences . . . difficulty in directing libido towards objects in outer reality. He becomes afraid to love" (1941, p. 50). The child is simply trying to love and to connect with the object. Repression would be unnecessary if only the object could tolerate that love. When Fairbairn criticizes Freud for focusing on depressive rather than schizoid problems, he is arguing for a shift in clinical emphasis away from the child's internal conflicts and toward conflicts with the object.

The Problem of Separation

A related problem emerges in the way relational theorists think about separation from the object. Fairbairn's one drive (libido) is unambivalently object-*seeking*. The same is true of Kohut's monistic need for the selfobject's acceptance of the emerging needs of the self. Within the terms of these theories, why would anyone ever move away from the object? One-drive theorists suggest two possibilities. First, there is withdrawal (schizoid in Fairbairn's terms, narcissistic in Kohut's) from traumatically bad relationships. Second, there is forced separation from a good object (either because of the object's unavailability or because of the intervention of some outside agency).

Basing his observations on this assumption, Fairbairn arrived at the following, sweeping conclusion: "separation from his object becomes the child's greatest source of anxiety" (1946, p. 145). Arnold Modell, whose sensibility has been shaped by Fairbairn's work as well as by Winnicott's and Kohut's, builds on Bowlby's (1969, 1973) ideas to suggest: "Separation of the infant and child from its mother results, in all primate species so far investigated, in a reaction of anxiety and what can be interpreted as grief" (1990, p. 188).

Fairbairn and Modell present what they have to say about separation as facts that should be evident to any observer. But they are not facts at all, or, to put it more accurately, they are facts drawn from an observational field already delimited by the theory. Certainly it is true that children react to separation with anxiety and grief in some circumstances. But at other times they do not. The child's reaction is entirely dependent on how and when the separation occurs. It is not separation per se that leads to anxiety and grief—only *premature* or *unwanted* separation. Phase-appropriate separation instigated by the child himself is a well-documented source of the sense of mastery and feelings of exuberance. This is true even when

the separation is accompanied or even provoked by disillusionment with the object.

Both Fairbairn and Modell assumed that the object is unambivalently needed as a source of security and as the supplier of the child's dependency needs. As a result, neither took account of separation motivated by the child's own needs. This leads us to a broader problem: what motivates the child (and later the adult) to move away from his objects? Clearly we all do this, even when the object has not failed us. The oscillating movement toward and away from others is an important dynamic current in all human experience. Fairbairn and Kohut can account for object seeking, but their one-drive theories cannot explain aversive reactions to and desire to separate from the good object.

Modell's theoretical vision shapes his clinical sensibility. Consistent with his ideas about separation, he interprets patients' attempts to establish distance as *defensive* reactions to failed relationships. Thus there is "a defense against relatedness" that takes the form of an "illusion of omnipotent self-sufficiency . . . a form of self-holding." Although it is defensive when it appears in the analysis, both the illusion and the self-holding originated as adaptive responses to "perceived failures in parental holding." Later in life, they serve to mask the "extent of the patient's dependency" (1990, pp. 192–193).

Certainly the phenomena Modell describes do occur often enough in any analyst's practice. My criticism is that his formulation leaves no room for nonrelatedness that is not defensive, or not responsive to relational inadequacy. Nonrelatedness for Modell is similar to resistance for Bacal: both are provoked by somebody's failure to respond appropriately. In sharp contrast, I believe that nonrelatedness and resistance are essential facets of all object relationships. To be effective, a drive theory must capture the aversive as well as the attractive features of our experience of other people.

Freud was so impressed by the inevitability of ambivalence—by our tendency to separate from as well as to approach other people—that he formulated four separate explanations of it.

1. Because of the workings of the death instinct, there is a natural pull away from relatedness and connection. This tendency affects not only human experience but life itself on every level. Organic material disintegrates into inorganic, cells break down, and social organizations (large groups and dyads alike) fragment.

2. The aggressive drive, a derivative of the death instinct, creates bad

objects, in the same way that libido creates good objects. We want to destroy the objects of our aggressive impulses, regardless of what the object has done to or for us.

3. Instinctual conflict makes all object relations unsatisfactory in some measure, regardless of what has happened in the relationship. Because incompatible impulses—transformations of desire and rage—are always directed toward the same object, frustration is inevitable. That we will be ambivalent about all relationships is one of the most clinically powerful implications of the dual-instinct theory.

4. Freud wrote that "something in the nature of the sexual instinct itself is unfavourable to the realization of complete satisfaction" (1912b, pp. 188–189). There are a number of reasons for this, but the one that best captured Freud was the idea that when the original component instincts are forged into a unified, "mature" sexual drive, a great deal of what originally seemed urgent is inevitably left behind. The diversity of pregenital desires means that no relationship will ever fully satisfy us.

Although its limitations are well documented, the libido/aggression theory captures the inherent paradox of human relatedness: there is frustration built into every satisfaction, and a satisfaction in every frustration as well. Our needs and passions drive us away from our objects even as they move us toward them. A great deal of this is lost in the drive theories of the relational model each of which, in its own way, suggests that we are moved by needs and desires that are ultimately satisfiable and offer the possibility of unambivalent relationships. Separation, in these theories, is evidence that there has been some failure, a breakdown in the normal order of things. The texture and complexity of Freud's insight into human intimacy cannot be supported by the drives of the relational model. In the next two chapters I will attempt to build a drive theory that preserves the intricacy of Freud's model without succumbing to its narrowness.

The Somatic Strategy

FREUD often said that his psychoanalytic vision was simultaneously directed inward, toward peoples' impulses, and outward, toward what has happened to them in their lives. Everybody wants to know whether neuroses are "the inevitable result of a particular constitution or the product of certain detrimental (traumatic) experiences in life." But we might as well ask, "Does a baby come about through being begotten by its father or conceived by its mother?" (1916–17, pp. 346–347). In fact, neither the neurosis nor the baby is possible without some contribution from both sides.

It is a nice clinical thought, this "complemental series," but not one that finds a great deal of support in Freud's own metapsychology. In the final analysis, because it is built on the dual-instinct theory, Freud's interpretive system focuses attention on the analysand's impulse life and directs us to impute sexual or aggressive aims to the impulses we discover or construct. Working with this theoretical foundation, analysts probing the unconscious assume that what they will find is the sexual or aggressive urge, not impressions of life's experiences.

A vignette will demonstrate how the assumptions of drive theory influence the analyst's interpretive posture. The case illustrates how the analyst is led to hear and interpret the impulse at the expense of all other possibilities, and also how the impulse itself is inevitably understood to derive from the workings of the sexual drive. It is drawn from a paper by Martin Silverman (1987), designed to provide clinical material for discussion by analysts of various theoretical persuasions.

Silverman's patient is a young woman who sought treatment for sexual and social inhibitions, masochistic tendencies, and depression. He reports

a history of "pseudostupidity" enacted with her father, evidently from early childhood to the present. I am going to focus my comments on a fantasy reported by the patient and on the analyst's interpretation of it. Leading up to the fantasy, the patient summarizes a number of situations she has described: "I get intimidated with men. I always feel that they know they have the knowledge. They have the brains, and I'm dumb . . . It's the same thing here. I keep feeling like asking you, 'What does it mean?' I always feel like you know . . . I feel you're always a step ahead of me. You *know*, because you're smarter than I am and all the training and experience you have." At this point the analyst intervenes: "I don't think that's what it is. I think you feel I know because I'm a man, that as a woman you don't have the brains." (pp. 152–153).

The patient talks a bit about men, including one who rejected her somewhat crudely, and also about being intimidated. She says she was intimidated at the hairdresser's, both by the man who cut her hair and by the woman who shampooed it and "put her fingers into my hair" (pp. 153–154). The analyst intervenes again to tell her that this description sounds sexual. The patient appears to demur but then describes a masturbation fantasy: "There's—a doctor—a mad scientist—and his nurse and—he ties me down to—do things to me . . . The fantasy had to do with—something—it had to do with getting bigger breasts. It's foolish—I feel sheepish [pause]. It's so silly [pause]." Again the analyst speaks: "There's nothing silly about it; you mobilize those feelings to push away and avoid looking into the fantasy and feelings" (p. 154).

The patient goes on, talking about her intimidation by men and returning to the fantasy. She becomes more explicit about a "slave and master" theme, refers to pornographic elements of it, and mentions bondage. She feels that she has to submit masochistically to the powerful men who have something to offer her but would enslave her in return. The analyst interprets the transferential aspect of the fantasy to the patient, concluding, "You want *me* to be the mad scientist forcing and hurting you and making changes in you" (p. 155).

In discussing the presentation, Gill accurately targets the problem in Silverman's interpretation. The crucial point is that Silverman tells the patient that she *wants him to be* the mad scientist rather than that she *experiences him* this way (1987, p. 251; see Levenson [1987] for a similar argument). Gill points out, and I certainly agree, that the patient would have good reason to believe that she was engaged, submissively and even masochistically, with a mad scientist who demands surrender as the price for what he has to offer.

Consider: even in my edited version of a brief segment of one hour, Silverman contradicts his patient twice. He tells her that she is wrong about why she feels he's smarter and that she doesn't really feel silly about describing her fantasy. He also comes up with an interpretation that may well strike the patient as coming from left field (the sexual meaning of having her hair washed and cut), and he has been quite insistent about it.

It does not matter much at the moment whether Silverman is right or wrong in his interpretation. More interesting is his immediate, apparently unquestioning assumption that his patient's fantasy reflects a transferential wish rather than a transferential impression. What is it about Silverman's version of psychoanalytic theory that supports or even requires this clinical perspective?

In my first chapter I argued that Freud turned his theory inexorably toward the assumption that unconscious contents are determined originally and primarily by endogenous forces. This is a vision rooted in the philosophical rationalism of Descartes and Leibniz; it prescribes a point of view from which drive analysts gather their clinical data, construct patterns in what they have seen, and formulate their interpretations. Silverman's approach to his patient strikes me as rationalism run amok.

Freud gave rationalism a particular twist. In his version the endogenous forces that shape experience are not originally of the mind; they arise within the body, acquiring psychological meaning only secondarily. This binds psychology inextricably to biology and traces behavior to its roots in our organismic endowment. When Hartmann wrote that "the foundation on which Freud built his theory of neurosis is not 'specifically human' but 'generally biological,'" he was stipulating that experience emerges from physiological processes (1939a, p. 28). Just as human nature, for Freud, precedes society and determines its organization, so our biological nature precedes and determines human psychology.

Freud's decision to construct psychoanalytic principles on a biological base represents one theoretical choice among many (Schafer, 1976). My purpose here will be to explore this decision with a view to determining whether the advantages claimed for it hold up to close scrutiny.* If the attempt to base the drives in somatic processes cannot be justified, we

---

*I will not address a further question that is of interest in its own right: which of the competing evolutionary/biological visions—there are many—can be most fruitfully applied to psychoanalytic thinking? Mitchell (1988) has discussed this on the basis of recent anthropological data that promote a revised view of human phylogeny. Friedman (1985) and Slavin (1985) also reconsider specific psychoanalytic hypotheses in light of alternative biological models.

must confront some challenging questions about Freud's rationalist interpretive system.

Was Freud a Biologist?

Discussions of the relation between psychoanalytic concepts and biological (especially neuroanatomical and neurophysiological) findings have been endlessly complicated by a long-standing ad hominem attack on Freud from authors who are dissatisfied with the structure of psychoanalytic theory. These authors have tried to move the theory away from its emphasis on the operation of somatically based drives that build tension and press for discharge according to the dictates of the constancy principle. Wanting to move the theory, they feel obliged to move Freud first; they have sought out (or constructed) constraints on his thinking that prevented him from fully appreciating the psychological implications of his own clinical work. Freud, they suggest, was so tied to his background in the laboratory that he could not see the psychological forest for the neurological trees. In constructing their particular version of Freud, they have drawn heavily on his academic background and on the theoretical ambitions that putatively grew from it, but their historical scholarship is the public face of doctrinal polemic. They have promoted a vision of Freud based on a partial excavation of the intellectual influences that guided him, and on an equally partial sampling of his early writings.

Their argument runs like this: Freud was a crypto-biologist who, following the lead of his most revered teachers, attempted to build a model of the mind on the basis of then current but now abandoned physiological principles. Freud was most influenced by the neuropsychiatrist Theodor Meynert and the physiologist Ernst Brücke, followers of the physicalist school of Helmholtz. Reacting against the popular, long-standing, but exhausted vitalist tradition, this group had sworn an oath (literally) to construct only physico-chemical explanations of organismic processes. Freud's continuing commitment to his mentors' vision deeply affected the direction of his theorizing. In a formulation that has been influential despite its extravagance, Siegfried Bernfeld wrote, "In spite of the new revolutionary features of psychoanalysis, its core is a continuation of the work that Freud did for Brücke" (1944, p. 356).

The argument continues: The *Project for a Scientific Psychology* (1895), never published, represents Freud's most explicit statement of his intentions. It is a kind of physicalist manifesto, applying then current "anti-

vitalist neurological dogma" to the workings of the mind (Holt, 1965b, p. 97). His first explicitly psychological model of the mind in chapter 7 of *The Interpretation of Dreams* simply translated the mechanisms of the *Project* into a new language (G. Klein, 1976). Freud's heart, and therefore his vision, remained with his physicalist mentors; psychology itself was nothing more than an intermediate stage to be tolerated until the organic substrate on which mind rested could be revealed. Psychic energies (libido, aggression, eros, the death instinct) are stand-ins for the physical energies that fuel the brain machine; psychic structures (ego, id, superego) are the parts of the machine. Freud's thinking about the workings of these energies and structures—his metapsychology—was never intended as a psychology at all, Gill argues (1976). Quite to the contrary, metapsychological principles are biological, inherently and by Freud's own design.

Proponents of the interpretation of Freud as what Sulloway has called a "biologist of the mind" (1979) are prominent in psychoanalytic circles; they have achieved considerable influence. Their reading, however, is oversimplified; it envisions a young Freud already committed to an established approach to neurophysiology and its relation to psychology, a commitment from which he never wavered over the course of half a century. They claim that his attempts to reduce psychological phenomena to the natural-science language of force and structure infiltrate his theory making from the beginning of his career to the end of his life.

The issue is more complex. Even to single out the unpublished *Project* as the best evidence for Freud's stand on the psychology/physiology relation early in his career is questionable and contentious.* Four years earlier he had published the monograph *On Aphasia* (1891), which was strongly influenced by the neurologist Hughling Jackson's theory of dynamic hierarchies. Jackson insisted that physical and psychical processes must be conceptualized separately and as parallel to each other. His vision was therefore antireductionist and antiphysicalist at its core. *On Aphasia,* unlike the *Project* explicitly a neurological work, changes our view of Freud's relationship to his laboratory instructors. Based on a Jacksonian model of the mind-brain relation, it can be aptly characterized as "a scathing attack upon the neurological theories of Freud's teachers" (Solms and Saling, 1986, p. 402; also Kanzer, 1973, 1983).

---

*The very question of whether Freud discarded the *Project* is hotly debated. Edelson (1984) and Solms and Saling (1986) among others believe that he did. Kanzer (1973) vigorously argues that he did not.

Attempts to understand Freud are thus confronted with a problem that is ignored by those who want to portray him simply as continuing the tradition of Helmholtz and Brücke. Freud was exposed to a range of positions on the relation between psychological and biological phenomena. There is no one neurological point of view that can be said to have influenced him most, and there is no one place in his writings where he expresses his own preferences explicitly. Most of the evidence suggests that his neurological views are best set forth in *On Aphasia,* but then how are we to read the apparently physicalist intentions of the *Project?* For many analysts the answer is to read it essentially as a psychology. Its foremost purpose is to conceptualize psychological observations through the metaphorical use of the language of neurophysiology.* Certainly Freud had grander theoretical ambitions too: in the opening sentence of the *Project* he declares that its purpose is "to represent psychical processes as quantitatively determinate states of specifiable material particles" (1895, p. 295). But as the argument of the manuscript develops, it does not appear that Freud was trying to explain psychological events simply as a function of known processes occurring in the brain. Quite the opposite. His aim was to construct a model of brain structure and function that could accommodate the clinical data, especially data drawn from his analysis of the flow of ideas in the defense neuroses. It is more likely, then, that the brain depicted in the *Project* is a heuristic embodiment of the neurotic mind than that the mind is a disembodied Helmholtzian brain.

Ultimately, neither the extent of Freud's neurophysiological ambitions nor the neurological principles that most significantly shaped his thinking can ever be known directly. Interpretations of his objectives are inevitably shaped by the commentator's own theoretical program. They can only be creatively (and, in the current state of psychoanalysis, tendentiously) reconstructed. In any case, to seek a theoretical guide in Freud's historical intentions is to fall into an intellectual version of the genetic fallacy. It serves Freud poorly to limit the scope of his theory to his original intentions for it. From the perspective of the practicing analyst, whether Freud based his psychology on a presumed biological substrate or whether he hoped some day to find one matters little. What psychoanalytic theory offers us, *as analysts,* is a psychology—regardless of its intellectual prove-

---

*Lustman (1968), Friedman and Alexander (1983), Kanzer (1973, 1983), Mancia (1983), Reiser (1985), Solms and Saling (1986), and in an especially well-reasoned article Parisi (1987) have argued this position.

nance. This does not of course rule out the possibility that it can also suggest possibilities to biologists.

The Drives and the Body

Whatever his intentions, Freud's particular application of philosophical rationalism was based in his vision of the relation between mind and body. When he argued that all psychic phenomena originate with the activity of endogenous stimuli, he meant that these stimuli impinge on the mind from within the body of the organism. This formulation has nothing to do with biological models of the mind itself or with actual or potential organic substrates. It addresses the *psychological* problem of what moves the mind and has a direct effect on the interpretive system of psychoanalysis, as illustrated by the vignette from Silverman.

Throughout his life, Freud believed that somatic stimuli have a special status in human psychology. These stimuli—experienced as urges or impulses—arise within the body as the result of physiological processes and operate as the prime movers of the mind, which itself comes into existence to make their satisfaction possible. Although this formulation is generally associated with the drive theory of psychoanalysis, it long predates the advent of the drive model. As early as the *Project* Freud found the intimate connection between mind and body to be the "*mainspring* of the psychical mechanism." Thus, he argues, "in the interior of the system there arises the impulsion which sustains all psychical activity" (1895, pp. 316, 317). In chapter 7 of *The Interpretation of Dreams,* Freud envisions a mind energized by wishes, which are desires to recreate experiences of satisfaction. Wishes arise when there is some homeostatic imbalance, most likely caused by a surge of "the major somatic needs" (1900, p. 565).

Freud's idea that the stimuli impinging upon the mind as motive forces originate within the body decisively influenced his construction of the drive concept itself. In his favorite definition, drive is a "demand made upon the mind for work in consequence of its connection with the body" (1915a, p. 122). And, detailing the distinguishing characteristics of drive, he defined its source as "the somatic process which occurs in an organ or part of the body" (p. 123). Almost two decades later, addressing the issue from the relatively new structural perspective, Freud envisioned an id that is "open at its end to somatic influences" (1933, p. 73). Finally, in his last attempt at a general theoretical statement in the *Outline of Psychoanalysis,* Freud reasserted his conviction: "There can be no question but that the

libido has somatic sources, that it streams to the ego from various organs and parts of the body" (1940, p. 151).

As Schur (1966) has pointed out, there was no psychological interpretation of the drives until long after Freud had discussed them biologically. Even the well-known idea that drive lies on the frontier between the psychic and the somatic first appears, somewhat incidentally, in the Schreber case (1911b, p. 74). The idea was not formally introduced into the metapsychology until 1915, in a passage added to the *Three Essays* (1905a, p. 168) and in "Instincts and Their Vicissitudes" (1915a, pp. 121–122). Psychoanalysis had been practiced and theorized about for more than twenty years (and a great deal of its conceptual structure was established in ways that have not yet been superseded) before there was any idea of drive as a psychological construct. And even then Freud insisted on its somatic origins.

Freud built psychoanalysis on the assumption that in the final analysis the body moves the mind. Organic stimuli energize the mind—quite literally, they "drive" it and therefore initiate and color all psychological experience. The aim of every instinct, Freud asserts, is "removing the state of stimulation at the source" (1915a, p. 122). It makes no psychological sense, theoretically or clinically, to ask why the stimulus has a particular quality—why, for example, a particular impulse requires sexual activity for its satisfaction. Thus: "excitations of two kinds arise from the somatic organs, *based upon differences of a chemical nature*. One of these kinds of excitation we describe as being specifically sexual" (1905a, p. 168, my italics). The quality of the stimulus depends on the somatic process. Ultimately, we reach a point where the need itself is psychologically irreducible—it cannot be further analyzed. I will call the line of argument embodied in these assumptions "the somatic strategy."

Freud's immediate followers working within the drive model all adopted the somatic strategy. It is an essential premise in the formulations of Hartmann (1939a), Loewenstein (1940), Kris (1947), and other leading figures of the first-generation ego psychologists. Fenichel, for example, considered it a fundamental assumption of psychoanalytic theory that "noninstinctual phenomena have to be explained as the effects of external stimuli on biological needs" (1945, p. 11). Contemporary proponents of the strategy do not generally feel obliged to articulate it explicitly, but there are exceptions. In a series of papers Compton has explicitly argued that it is essential to retain a view of drive based on the idea that "certain physiologic processes which commence . . . outside of the central

nervous system have a special relation to psychological phenomena" (1983, p. 373).

Even when the somatic strategy is not explicitly argued, it continues implicitly to determine much of the contemporary use of the concepts "drive," "libido," and (more controversially) "aggression." Joseph Sandler, for example, includes drive among the "influences arising from within the body" (1972, p. 296; also Sandler and Joffe, 1965, 1966). And Fred Pine, in the context of a theoretical approach aimed at a considerable broadening of the traditional drive model, lists as one of the "defining features of psychoanalysis" the idea that "bodily based experiences of drive and gratification" are central components of mental life (1985, p. 71).

It is essential to my argument, here and throughout the book, that the somatic strategy is in fact only a strategy. It is a theoretical option, not an a priori necessity in building psychoanalytic theory (as Pine would have it), and certainly not an empirical discovery generated by the psychoanalytic method. It is possible to accept the idea of a drive (defined as an endogenous prime mover of the mind) without granting the drives unique somatic or psychosomatic status. The earliest arguments along these lines that I have been able to find appear, in remarkably similar terms, in the work of Jeanne Lampl-de Groot (1956) and Samuel Novey (1957). Hardly revisionist in their views of mental dynamics, both authors maintain that the value of the dual-instinct theory lies only in its psychological implications. Both suggest that any correlation between the drives as clinical phenomena and their putative biological origins adds nothing to our understanding of mental activity.

In contemporary discussion, the attempt to separate drive as a psychological concept from any special connection with a somatic source has been most closely associated with the work of Charles Brenner (1980b, 1982). His argument, and the very similar position of Arthur Valenstein (in Panel, 1968), is that while all mental phenomena can be presumed to have a somatic base (because mental functioning requires brain functioning), the drives have neither a unique relationship to an organic source nor a distinctive location on a psychosomatic "frontier."

Brenner believes that the drives must be regarded as purely psychological phenomena because they are based on purely psychological data, the observations of working psychoanalysts. "Each observation," he writes, "is that of a particular person's wish for a particular kind of gratification from a particular person, under particular circumstances." On the basis of many analyses, certain generalizations are possible. "One of these is that such

wishes fall readily into two broad groups, sexual and aggressive . . . these generalizations are expressed succinctly by the psychoanalytic theory of the drives" (1980a, pp. 209, 210).

A position that is aesthetically and epistemologically remote from Brenner's but that shares much of its psychological sensibility (and some of its problems) has been advanced by Roy Schafer. In Schafer's view, patients present themselves for analysis with particular narrative versions of their life histories. Much of the analytic process consists of patient and analyst reconstructing these narratives in a way that allows the patient to experience a deeper and ultimately more benign version of the experience. The analyst's role is not (as it is for Brenner) simply to observe and to generalize. Rather, from the beginning the analyst "follows certain storylines of personal development, conflictual situations, and subjective experience that are the distinguishing features of his or her analytic theory and approach" (1983, p. 187). Drive is one such storyline. Others include Kohut's cohesive self, Klein's rageful infant at the breast, and Mahler's infant moving toward separation and individuation.

Schafer strongly endorses the interpretive implications of the dual-instinct theory: "As analysts we are always concerned to view actions in terms of infantile psychosexual and aggressive conflicts and the variations of these that the analysand has continued to fashion along with a suitable environment in which to enact them" (p. 91). In an apparent paradox, though, he rejects the storyline embodied by drive in another sense: he objects to the vision of a "passive self being driven by internal forces." This he sees simultaneously as facilitating disclaimed responsibility and as moralistic (p. 225). It would seem that Schafer objects to the biological elements of the drive storyline, while continuing to hold its psychological lessons. He objects to the idea that drive—and thus all motives—originate somatically. This, he believes, promotes disclaimers that one is being "lived by" one's body. Similarly, it supports moralistic pseudo-interpretations that pressure patients to renounce or sublimate primitive impulses.

One effect of Schafer's reconstruction of psychoanalytic investigation and theory making has been to free the drive concept from its biological roots. In this sense, although he has approached the problem from an entirely different set of assumptions than Brenner, he reaches similar psychological (but not epistemological) conclusions.

THE WORK of the authors just discussed makes it clear that the somatic strategy is debatable in contemporary psychoanalysis. None of these authors, however, gives adequate credit to the fact that it is not merely quix-

otic to insist on the somatic roots of drives (viewed as prime movers of the mind). There are some good reasons, from the point of view of theoretical coherence, for retaining the somatic strategy. First, the strategy accounts for the peremptory, "driven" experience of certain needs; second, it solves the vexing problem of how to confirm psychoanalytic hypotheses about the nature of human motivation; and third, it addresses the need to have a complete (psychosomatic) theory of the human organism.

In the end I don't see any of these reasons as convincing enough, but they must be acknowledged. I will devote the rest of this chapter to presenting the arguments in favor of the somatic strategy, along with my rejoinders to each. Some of the rejoinders I think are decisive; others are admittedly inconclusive and raise more questions than they answer. My goal is to show that the somatic strategy is not inevitable and is not even the best choice among those available. I hope my discussion will pave the way to a fresh look at the drive concept, a look based on its interpretive implications freed from the constraints of the shotgun marriage of psychology and biology.

The somatic source of the drives is necessary to account for the urgency of certain needs. These needs underlie behaviors that we think of as "driven," and these behaviors are of crucial interest to psychoanalysts.

In his review of the psychoanalytic theory of motivation, Rapaport insisted that peremptoriness is one of the defining characteristics of the drive concept (1960, p. 865). Freud's interest in peremptoriness was an inevitable consequence of his attempt to account for neurotic symptoms. By definition, symptoms are ego-dystonic and have a compulsive quality; the triumph of hysterical incapacity or obsessive-compulsive ritual over conscious will was Freud's model phenomenon in need of explanation. His question was how can behaviors that are so patently maladaptive become so compelling to the neurotic? His answer was that driven behaviors are motivated by urgent needs, which originate in and reflect characteristics of the body. Our experience of bodily stimuli, Freud wrote at the very end of his life, "exercise a more peremptory influence on our mental life than external perceptions" (1940, p. 161).

Contemporary supporters of the somatic strategy follow a similar line. Allan Compton has written that the "special relation" of the drives to their physiological origins "is intended to account for . . . driven-ness. Something essential would seem to be lost by eliminating this relationship as an integral factor in the explanatory construct of drives" (1983, p. 373). Marshall Edelson defines an instinctual wish as "the sign of a hypothetical

central state or process in a biological system," and uses the definition to account for the peremptoriness, persistence, and recurrence of these wishes (1984, p. 97). Benjamin Rubinstein, who rejects traditional accounts of the somatic origin of the drives, warns that in divorcing motive from the body we lose the ability to account for the impelling nature of certain needs (in Brenner, 1980b).

There are two important objections to the argument that the explanation of driven behavior requires a somatic source of drive. I will spell these out in some detail, not only because they are interesting in their own right but because each has significant clinical implications. The somatic strategy is no mere metapsychological wrinkle; it has a direct impact on the interpretive posture of the working analyst.

My first objection to the somatic strategy focuses on the definition of what is considered peremptory in the first place. What does a psychoanalyst really mean when he writes, as if the referent were self-evident, of "the importunacy of many kinds of driven behavior" (Holt, 1967a, p. 37)? Many approaches rely on a strikingly narrow perspective. This will become clear if we pause for a moment to take a look at what needs people typically feel driven to satisfy. Probably the first to come to mind are those clearly tied to somatic requirements: the nearly constant need for oxygen, the need to drink when thirsty, the need to urinate when the bladder is full (the need that Holt, 1976, says comes closest to fitting the model of drive theory), and so on. If the somatic strategy is designed to explain peremptoriness, why aren't these considered among the fundamental drives? In fact they once were—under the heading of the ego or self-preservative instincts. But Freud never believed that studying the neuroses would illuminate the workings of such drives, and eventually he dropped them from his dual-instinct theory.

There are many reasons for Freud's relative lack of interest in the ego instincts, but certainly one is that they are *too* peremptory. Their satisfaction tolerates no (or at most very little) delay, and their aim and object are genetically fixed. In Freud's terms, they are not subject to vicissitudes; in the more contemporary language of George Klein (1976), they lack "plasticity." So they cannot lie at the root of the convoluted and conflicted attempts at gratification that characterize neurosis.

This line of thought reveals a substantial logical flaw in the somatic strategy: the somatic origin of the drives is held necessary to account for needs that are peremptory, but there are some needs that are too peremptory (and in a sense too somatic) to be accorded a fundamental role in the structure of psychoanalytic theory.

But an even more interesting problem emerges when we take a broader look at human development across the life cycle. There is, perhaps, a more subversive question: how peremptory, in the long run, is sexual or aggressive discharge? Certainly orgasm feels urgent in a highly stimulated person, and an angry reaction may feel imperative to someone who has been insulted, thwarted, or punished. But these events take as their frame of reference only isolated moments in a lifetime. Thinking about life histories as the psychoanalyst does leads to a very different vision of what is most imperative—we are likely to come up with a wide range of answers when we ask ourselves what is most urgent to a particular patient. What I have in mind may include getting away from home, avoiding risks, being creative, leading an unexceptional life, avoiding publicity, achieving power, providing a better life for one's children. These needs are certainly less closely tied to somatic processes than sexual arousal and discharge. They are not, on this account, less urgent in the conduct of an individual life, either as that life is subjectively experienced or as it is observed and constructed by the analyst. By what warrant, then, are these urgent aims reduced to the apparently unrelated aims of sexual and aggressive discharge, especially when those are not themselves our most peremptory organic needs?

This problem has been addressed by various authors who agree on very little except that a range of human motives, many of them far removed from any connection with a somatic source, exercise a more peremptory influence on human growth and development than sexual and aggressive discharge do. In an incisive paper, Apfelbaum traces objections to the limited definition of peremptory needs back to Erikson's work. Because he "consistently transcends any distinction between ego and drive," Apfelbaum argues, Erikson is able to demonstrate just how compelling a range of motives can be (1966, p. 459). These include the need to synthesize (Erikson, 1963) and strivings for independence, mastery, and exploration (Erikson, 1943). On the basis of his observations of very young infants, Daniel Stern has reached conclusions quite similar to Erikson's. Referring to his subjects' exploration, curiosity, search for cognitive novelty, and pleasure in mastery, Stern concludes that a wide range of different motives move the child, all of which "are backed by some imperative" (1985, p. 238).

In his broad recasting of psychoanalytic motivational theory, Joseph Sandler has taken a similar approach to the problem of peremptoriness:

an essential element in intrapsychic conflict is what can be called the *unconscious peremptory urge*. By "peremptory" in this context I mean that quality of

compellingness and urgency, of being "automatic," of being driven by a force, which we usually associate with instinctual wishes or their more direct derivatives. However, this so-called peremptory tendency is not confined to the id, but may be regarded as a function of various aspects of the apparatus (1974, p. 53).

Later Sandler specified the quality of "peremptory impulses," including among them "urges to actualize . . . quite complicated wishful fantasies" (Sandler and Sandler, 1983, p. 418). These fantasies may or may not involve physiologically based needs; in any case, their urgency is unrelated to the discharge of bodily tensions.

Erikson, Stern, and Sandler, each in his own way, have loosened the tie between the peremptoriness of motives and any assumption of a somatic source. Each describes motives that, despite their urgency, cannot be traced to organic events. Each builds his case for peremptoriness on purely psychological grounds, thereby avoiding the limitations of the somatic strategy.

Let me summarize the argument to this point. Freud was concerned with the peremptoriness of certain needs because he was attempting to understand the compulsive quality of neurotic symptoms. His assumptions about the openness of the mind to somatic stimuli led him to explain peremptoriness on the basis of the mind-body connection. But this narrow focus limited his vision in two ways: he was not able to integrate the most peremptory, most obvious bodily needs into his system because these were not implicated in the neuroses; and he was not able to see the broader developmental imperatives that are most urgent in the formation of personality and of "nonsymptomatic" character pathology.

A SECOND objection to the somatic explanation of driven behavior focuses on the way adherents of the somatic strategy take their patients' reports of peremptory urges and their enactment of driven behavior at face value. These analysts assume that the origin of psychological urgency lies in a quantitative increase: when the accumulation of stimulus reaches a threshold level, some form of discharge is necessary. Subjectively, at certain levels of stimulus intensity, the behaviors that serve the discharge function will be experienced as imperative or driven. This formulation reflects the workings of the constancy principle and the operation of a mind impinged upon by somatic stimuli.

It can be tempting to formulate theory in a way that closely reflects patients' self-appraisals. But, as Schafer has pointed out, the self-appraisals

themselves require psychological explanation and must not be taken as the last word (1983, p. 225). *Feeling* driven by one's body is not the same as *being* driven.

A brief example will show how the experience of drivenness neither requires nor supports the somatic strategy. A man in his thirties, living relatively contentedly in a long-standing homosexual relationship that was sexually satisfying, periodically felt compelled to pick up a strange man for a quick sexual encounter. He would start by going to a gay bar, move on to seedy bookstores or movie theaters, and (if unsuccessful at finding someone, which he usually was) would wind up with a prostitute. The search typically lasted for many hours. During this time he would feel a constantly escalating urgency focused on the imagined moment of orgasm. His thoughts were concentrated exclusively on the fantasied encounter, time passed quickly, his heart pounded. Although at first he had a particular sort of man in mind, as the night went by he became less and less focused on his partner; only the orgasm itself mattered. When he finally connected with somebody, the result was invariably disappointing; he was marginally able to achieve and maintain an erection and the orgasm itself was only more or less intense. As soon as it was over he would feel guilty, ashamed, and depressed. The dysphoria always lasted for a day or two. Although he remembered his disappointment and self-loathing clearly, it never prevented him from repeating the pattern.

The contrast between this sexual behavior and the experience with his lover was striking. They had sex frequently, and while the anticipation was never so exciting as when he was cruising, the result was far better. He had no trouble with potency, orgasm was powerful, and he felt affectionate toward his lover after intercourse.

Prior to analysis, this patient had arrived at a conventional explanation of his behavior: he was oversexed, could not contain his impulses within the framework of a monogamous relationship, and so periodically experienced an irresistible impulse that he then acted out. His explanation, and the behavioral pattern itself, conforms to the vision of peremptory behavior held by proponents of the somatic strategy. Notice particularly the loosening of his criteria for an acceptable partner as the night wore on. Quantitative hypotheses derived from the somatic strategy predict that, as drive tension increases, more and more people will be experienced as appropriate sexual objects.

But consider what this account does not explain. It says nothing about why there should be such a buildup of tension in a man for whom sex was

easily available and satisfying. It says nothing about why he chose cruising over sex with his lover, knowing that the latter would be more gratifying. And it is circular: it assumes that the aim of the patient's behavior was sexual discharge and therefore ends the story with the sexual encounter itself. The patient's self-recriminations of the next day, and his disappointment in the sex itself, are interpreted as expectable (if perhaps somewhat harsh) superego reactions to having yielded to his impulses.

I tend to doubt that orgasm was the aim of this repetitive behavior. The patient's experience of his compulsive pattern fits well with the tendencies to self-derogation and disclaimed responsibility that Schafer sees as essential to the storyline of drivenness. Work with this man resulted in altering his own sense of the goal of his behavior: he experienced the aim of his cruising not as having sex but as having degraded sex, and therefore in the service of constructing a specific, quite familiar, although consciously unpleasant sense of himself and the conditions in which he lived. He saw himself as out of control sexually; this condemned him to banishment from the "normal" world of affectionate acceptance represented by his lover. He was part of a different world, a netherworld of desperate characters living on the fringe. His forays into their world—his membership in it—disgusted him, but the disgust was highly erotic too. Once he could see all this and gained a new understanding of what he was after, his associations moved quickly and relatively easily to the life-historical experiences on which the behavior was based.

In this analysis, and I think quite generally, the behaviors that felt most peremptory did not express a quantitative increase in motive strength. Rather, they derived from the most conflicted aspects of the patient's self-image and object relations. They were experienced as peremptory precisely because they were conflicted; the conflict itself was expressed in the impulsive quality of the actions. The somatic strategy guides us away from this clinically useful implication of conflict theory and toward a view based on primitive notions about the accumulation of quantities of stimulus. In this formulation I agree with the arguments of Kubie (1947) and Apfelbaum (1962) that the illusory simplicity of quantitative explanations can mask the true goals and therefore the meaning of behavior.

Positing a somatic source of the drives solves an important scientific problem of psychoanalysis. It points the way to confirming fundamental interpretive hypotheses without relying on unreliable psychological data.

In a passage from "Instincts and Their Vicissitudes," Freud addressed

the epistemological problems of psychoanalysis in a striking way. Having spelled out, quite tentatively, the dual-instinct theory, he went on to raise the question of how we know that these are the most fundamental human needs. His answer:

> I am altogether doubtful whether any decisive pointers for the differentiation and classification of the instincts can be arrived at on the basis of working over the psychological material. This working-over seems rather itself to call for the application to the material of definite assumptions concerning instinctual life, and it would be a desirable thing if those assumptions could be taken from some other branch of knowledge and carried over to psychology (1915a, p. 124).

Having said this, Freud immediately appealed to biology—specifically to the opinion of some biologists that "the sexual function differs from other bodily processes in virtue of a special chemistry" (p. 125). He recognized the difficulty of confirming fundamental interpretive assumptions within the clinical situation. The interpretive system itself, he suggested, infiltrates the collection and organization of data. But the somatic strategy would free psychoanalysis of its epistemological weakness.

The confirmation problem is still with us, and the somatic strategy is invoked as its solution. Consider the position of Robert Holt, who believes that the current state of psychoanalysis as a discipline "is not hopeless, but it *is* grave. We have been living in a fool's paradise, believing that our clinical theory was soundly established when in fact very little of it has been" (1985, p. 297). It is necessary for analysts to "listen to the neurophysiologist and his brethren in the laboratories, [so that] we can hope to avoid the presently besetting fault of psychoanalytic theory—its vagueness and untestability" (1967c, p. 532). Reviving the somatic strategy as a solution to our epistemological difficulties, Holt calls for development of "an intermediary or Janusian model . . . with one face turned towards biology, one towards psychology" (1981, p. 140).

A position closely related to Holt's has been adopted by Benjamin Rubinstein. Rubinstein argues against the possibility of testing broad psychoanalytic principles (the assumptions embodied in the dual-instinct theory would be a good example) in the clinical setting. Confirmation must come from extraclinical sources, especially neurophysiology. Rubinstein does not follow the traditional route of the somatic strategy in postulating a physiological source of drives. Instead he adopts a variant of the strategy, holding that all psychoanalytic concepts must be "protoneurophysiologi-

cal." That is, they must, at least in principle, be reducible to a physiological referent. Theoretical propositions must be confirmed "clinically, but also neurophysiologically. Only if they are confirmed in both of these ways can they . . . be truly explanatory" (1967, p. 66; also 1976). Rubinstein substitutes a conceptual connection between body and mind for the empirical, sequential connection suggested by Freud. Where Freud believed that the confirmation problem was addressed by placing the *origin* of the drives in the body, Rubinstein offers a contemporary version of the somatic strategy by requiring a physiological *referent* for all psychological constructs.

Authors who reject the somatic strategy cannot appeal to the physiologist to validate psychoanalytic hypotheses. What, then, happens to the confirmation problem in their hands? Generally it is either ignored or treated trivially. Brenner, for one, recognizes the problem, but consider his solution: "It was prudent in 1915 to be modest, even skeptical about the importance and reliability of purely psychoanalytic evidence, especially when used as a basis for drawing conclusions about the nature of the very wellsprings of human motivation. The same skepticism is not necessary today" (1982, p. 23). What, we may ask, has changed? Whatever evolves in any science, Brenner would reply; we have accumulated data that confirm some hypotheses and disconfirm others. Thus, "the evidential basis for psychoanalytic drive theory is the conscious and unconscious wishes of patients as disclosed by the psychoanalytic method of observation" (p. 21). And, "One need not hesitate . . . to base a theory of drives on psychoanalytic data, despite Freud's reluctance to do so himself" (1982, p. 20; also 1980a, pp. 209–210).

Brenner's position is based on a vision of "scientific" investigation that flourished in the nineteenth century and was codified by the logical positivists early in the twentieth. Roughly the position runs as follows: The "objective" observer approaches naked data, discovers certain "facts," and builds theories to explain those facts. As the levels of theoretical generalization and abstraction increase, the theories get further from the data, but their basis remains in the objectively observable facts. A straightforward application of this approach to the structure of psychoanalytic theory, which has been inexplicably and unfortunately persuasive to many analysts, was suggested by Robert Waelder (1962). For Waelder, the theorist begins with observations and moves from there through levels of abstraction including clinical interpretation, generalization, and theory, until one finally arrives at metapsychology.

The problem of course is that no investigator could ever even begin to

observe without certain guiding assumptions. This should be apparent to analysts as it is to few other investigators: it dovetails with the drive theory itself. Assumptions not only direct inquiry but even determine what is taken to be a fact, much as for Freud needs give our experience of external objects its particular meaning. Typically, however, analysts have not applied this to their own theory making. It has been left to philosophers to point out that each of us will reject the report of a fact out of hand if the fact is too discrepant with our theoretical assumptions about the world. David Hume remarked that this explains why we don't give much credit to reports of miracles (cited in Fodor, 1981). We may have similar reactions to such relatively commonplace phenomena as reported citings of flying saucers and data supporting parapsychological phenomena. Within psychoanalysis, Arnold Goldberg has given this a nice clinical twist: "One cannot expect to see a selfobject transference unless and until one believes in its existence" (1988, p. x).

Although Freud could be ambiguous on the point—he frequently, somewhat wistfully, describes the unclouded vision of the unbiased scientist—his formal statements are steeped in awareness of the contribution of the prepared mind of the investigator. The opening passage of "Instincts and Their Vicissitudes" is a model of caution: "Even at the stage of description it is not possible to avoid applying certain abstract ideas to the material in hand, ideas derived from somewhere or other but certainly not from the new observations alone" (1915a, p. 117). The concept of drive is just such an abstraction. Drive, Freud knew, does not simply emerge from the data. Rather, it figures importantly in the creation of the data, although the fruitfulness of psychoanalytic inquiry depends on the choice of an apt starting place. Despite Brenner's assertions, no discipline can prove its own postulates. Freud's attempt to circumvent this problem found expression in the somatic strategy.

It bears mentioning that while the difficulty of proving fundamental assumptions is a problem for all disciplines, it is particularly acute for psychoanalysis. Especially in the clinical setting, the hypotheses of the investigator influence the behavior of the subject, and this happens *by design*. Therapeutic goals—without which there would be no psychoanalytic situation in the first place—affect data at the most basic level. Considering the discrepancy between therapeutic goals and attempts to confirm theory, John Klauber wrote that thinking of the clinical setting as a laboratory "leaves a certain sense of unreality" (1968, p. 183). Adolf Grünbaum's (1984) bombastic critique of the claimed validity of psychoanalytic prop-

ositions, focused on the contaminating effect of suggestion, essentially re-states Klauber's point. Brenner is guilty of wishful thinking in arguing that existing clinical evidence adequately confirms the fundamental hypotheses of psychoanalysis.

Aware of the dilemma, Roy Schafer, another leading opponent of the somatic strategy, has taken a different, but no more successful, approach to the confirmation problem. Unlike Brenner, Schafer recognizes and rejects the positivist bias of much psychoanalytic theorizing. "There can be no theory-free and method-free facts," he writes, and his account of drive as a storyline fits that epistemological stance (1983, p. 188). But the storyline model can only defer, not avoid, the confirmation problem. Thus Schafer arrives at the following: "It does not follow . . . that all strategies of interpretation . . . have an equal claim on our attention and respect . . . I believe that it can be shown (though it would take extended discussion to make this demonstration), that some of these strategies are more penetrating, coherent, comprehensive *and mutative* than others" (p. 203, my italics). Indeed the discussion would be extended, but it is also necessary and Schafer never attempts it—this despite his conviction that the dual-instinct theory constitutes a preferred storyline; he reminds us repeatedly that analysis is most effective when the patient's life is constructed in terms of repetitive enactments of conflicted, infantile sexual and aggressive desires. This preference lands Schafer in the same confirmation muddle as everybody else; in cutting himself off from the somatic strategy he too has lost one apparent way out.

Neither decreeing that the confirmation problem has been solved nor sidestepping it by focusing on narrative standards serves psychoanalysis well. Admittedly this leaves psychoanalysis in an uncomfortable position, since there is no consensus that any of its most important hypotheses have been satisfactorily validated. But any number of authors have offered programs for doing so that both rely on purely psychological data and that use validational criteria as stringent as those of any science. Some (Edelson, 1984) believe that the clinical situation provides an adequate setting for the work of validation, while others (Wallerstein, 1976) do not. Among those who find extraclinical methodologies necessary, some work with the data of actual analytic hours (Weiss, Sampson, et al., 1986), while others rely on analog studies (Fisher and Greenberg, 1978; Silverman, Lachmann, and Milich, 1982). Although a great deal of this work has been interesting, nothing that has come out of it is conclusive. The situa-

tion is disturbing, but continuing efforts convince me that foreclosing the possibility of psychological confirmation, as Eagle (1980, p. 317) does, is premature.

Pointing out the ambiguity of psychological findings, advocates of the somatic strategy hold that validation is possible *only* if psychoanalytic theoretical constructs have an organic referent. But skepticism is not a proprietary commodity, and I would suggest that somatic strategists from Freud to the present have simply been asking too much of physiology. Physiological data can describe brain processes; they illuminate the generation and vicissitudes of neural stimuli. But mental activity is, by definition, not organic, and meaning as a concept has only a mental referent. There is nothing in physiological data that can, even in principle, address the hierarchy of meaning that psychoanalytic theory needs to confirm its hypotheses about "basic motivations."

Even if physiology were able to supply evidence of irreducible neural events that correlated perfectly with experienced motivational states, it is extremely unlikely that these events could be hierarchically ordered without considering psychological data. At the very end of his life, Freud came to believe that whatever we might learn about the brain will "give us no help towards understanding" mental life (1940, p. 145). The confirmation argument for the somatic strategy fails on the grounds that physiological reduction can never provide the evidence that the psychological theory of drive requires. Edelson has something similar in mind when he points to the difficulty of claiming that "it is [not] even possible for a proposition about the mind and a proposition about the brain to contradict each other . . . Efforts to tie psychoanalytic theory to a neurobiological foundation . . . should be resisted as expressions of logical confusion" (1984, p. 110).

The drives must have a somatic source because all behavior demonstrably involves bodily as well as mental activity. If psychoanalysis is ever to become a complete science of man, it must have a theory of motivation that is based upon and can account for the crossover between organic and mental events.

The somatic strategy is a specification of a broader point of view holding that any "complete" psychology must be a psychosomatic theory. This has been argued repeatedly by Rubinstein, for example in his statement that "behavior is bodily movement. It is implausible that mind can directly influence the body, bypassing brain . . . the effector structures are not mentalistic but neurophysiological structures" (1967, p. 65). A complete

understanding of behavior and experience therefore requires an under-standing of the sequence of organismic events. Psychoanalytic proposi-tions can be useful only if they cast light on that sequence.

Holt applied Rubinstein's general principle to a critique of the psycho-analytic theory of sexuality: "Surely the mind is not disembodied; sex, for example, is ineluctably a biochemical, anatomical, physiological, even genic matter, as well as one of conscious and unconscious meanings . . . to try to build up a systematic and comprehensive understanding of sexual behavior with this restriction seems to me false to Freud's example and his ambition for psychoanalysis" (1975, pp. 568–569). Expanding this point some years later, Holt charged: "Advocates of psychoanalysis as a 'pure psychology' would have us eliminate from our purview all bodily phe-nomena including psychosomatic symptoms, all hormonal, pharmaceuti-cal, and other biochemical influences on mood, thought, and behaviour, and any other direct consequences of the fact that we all have bodies" (1981, p. 136).

Morris Eagle (1980, 1984) has developed a similar argument from a slightly different starting point. He is highly impressed by a statement of Max Black's (1967, p. 656) that "as soon as reasons for action have been provided, an enquiring mind will want to press on to questions about the provenance and etiology of such reasons" (quoted by Eagle, 1980, p. 320). The search for the etiology of motives, Eagle believes, leads inex-orably to our organismic nature. Any full understanding of human desires, meanings, beliefs, or goals—any complete psychology—rests ultimately on "explanation in terms of 'purposeless' physical conditions and pro-cesses" (p. 313). We have all had bodies, *been* bodies, before we acquired minds. Throughout his paper and in his book, Eagle suggests that motives are little more than rationalizations; we construct them when the real forces driving us are beyond our grasp.*

The problem with this line of argument for the somatic strategy is not that it is untrue, but that it is based on a misleading premise and is there-fore irrelevant. Certainly no analyst would quarrel with the observation

---

*For example, Eagle argues that if we could arrange to stimulate a person's hypothalamus without his knowing it (a stimulation known to be associated with aggression), the person would come up with explanations of his anger based on his life circumstances. These expla-nations would rationalize the angry feeling, but they do not address its true (chemical, as Eagle would have it) cause. In a similar vein, Eagle reports on the "masculine" characteristics and preferences of women whose mothers had been given an androgen-related hormone during pregnancy (Money and Ehrhardt, 1972), discounting the relevance of "specific rea-sons and motives" these women would offer for their tendencies (pp. 327–329).

(actually quite trivial) that human life is a psychosomatic process. But the implication is precisely that no one discipline can provide the "comprehensive understanding" of behavior and experience that Holt finds necessary. Consider Holt's own enumeration of the factors affecting sexual behavior: he refers not only to biochemical, anatomical, physiological, and genic processes but also to influences deriving from "legal, institutional, cultural, economic, and even political" forces (1975, p. 569). Clearly the psychoanalytic contribution to the study of human sexuality is partial—but it is not on that account either incoherent or contingent. All disciplines have a partial contribution to make.

This observation is true generally. In fact, as far as I know, there is no such thing as a comprehensive theory of *anything*—baseballs, pineapples, or planets. Instead there is a range of theories to account for particular classes of observations, each class of observation being the province of a particular discipline. One could ask what discipline provides a comprehensive theory of the behavior of a baseball? That is, what discipline has a theory to account for what will happen to the baseball when it is dropped out of a window; what will happen when it falls into a vat of hydrochloric acid; what will happen when it is picked off the ground by an infielder after being hit to him during a game. Each of these situations poses different sets of circumstances, requiring specialized knowledge for the formulation of a reasonable hypothesis.

Explaining why a particular pitch was hit for a home run requires knowledge, grossly, of the data and hypotheses of physics, meteorology, physiology, and psychology (social and clinical), not to say baseball strategy. Information from each discipline accumulates gradually. Integration is unlikely to come from specialists in any one discipline; if it comes at all it will be the work of generalists. The difficulty of integrating disparate approaches is reflected in the weakness of predictive power: nobody can say with much confidence what will happen next in a baseball game. Campaigning for a "science of baseballs" that will be responsible for the overall coordination of human knowledge about the baseball as an object is an exercise in futility.

This is true, a fortiori, about something as complex as human behavior. Advocates of the somatic strategy fail to realize that every discipline has partial theories because every discipline is bound by its data. The data of psychoanalysis are the behaviors and experiences of patients as these unfold within the clinical setting. Edelson puts it this way: "We are not . . . directly studying a physiological system or an organism as a physical body,

and there is an important difference between the state of that system or body and the perception the subject has of its state. Even though the two are causally connected, they are not identical" (1984, p. 97).

Psychoanalytic inquiry into the "provenance and etiology" of motives—any inquiry into anything—must be limited by its method of inquiry and by its data. The analyst looking into the origin of experience and meanings finds only more of the same. Analytic explanations, therefore, are expressed in constructed patterns of experiences and meanings. Recognizing the incompleteness of these explanations must not lead analysts to bail out of a psychoanalytic approach into a biological one (or a social-psychological one, or to one based in any other discipline). This would amount to an abandonment of our own responsibilities as a field of inquiry. Advocates of the somatic strategy think we should stop being psychoanalysts and start being biologists as soon as we are confronted with an especially difficult problem.

Certainly there are fruitful lines of investigation into human experience that consider psychosomatic data and that work conceptually at the intersection of organic and mental processes. Along with many others, I expect that these lines of investigation will be the source of important advances in our understanding of human behavior and experience. Psychoanalysis can contribute to the evolving discipline of psychosomatic studies, but it *is not* that discipline; we have neither the data nor the methods.

The somatic strategy embodies what Edelson has aptly termed the "hegemonic" ambitions of some psychoanalytic theorists—a group that surely includes Freud. At the same time, however, the strategy weakens psychoanalytic theory itself by appealing to alternative sources of data when our own explanations seem inadequate. Advocates of the somatic strategy simultaneously ask too much and too little of psychoanalysis as a discipline.

Internal versus Biological

My arguments against the somatic strategy lead me to suggest a distinction that, as far as I know, has not been made in the psychoanalytic literature. It is the distinction between the psychological concept of an internal or endogenous force and the organismic concept of a "bodily" or "endosomatic" force. Consider, as an instance of the frequent confusion, Holt's use of "changes in the constituents of the blood" as an example of "internally generated contributions to motivation" (1967b, p. 87n). These

changes, clearly, are bodily, but in what sense are they psychologically internal?

It is a major argument running through this book that the most effective psychoanalytic theories work with a developed concept of endogenous processes. But my idea of the "endogenous" assumes (in contrast to the assumption of advocates of the somatic strategy) that psychoanalysis is a psychological theory. Thus the domain of psychoanalysis is the mind, and the endogenous is, by definition, mental. However one construes the endlessly debatable relationship between mind and body, it is also a matter of definition that bodily forces are not of the mind: the somatic is external to the mind.

There is no question, of course, that people have experiences (thirst comes to mind) and even behave (drinking comes to mind) in response to demonstrable somatic events, which can reasonably be considered to act as stimuli. But these stimuli cannot, again by definition, be endogenous determinants of behavior, since they are not endogenous to the mind. In fact, for a somatic stimulus to be a stimulus it must first be the object of experience (not necessarily conscious experience). This implies that it has already been interpreted by a mind whose purpose is to interpret sensory data. And that is an active mind—a mind that interprets all sensory data (endosomatic and exosomatic) in its own way. Gill has put a similar idea this way: "the body does not influence the psyche as such but only as it is psychologically represented" (1983a, p. 528; also Edelson, 1984, p. 97).

The distinction between psychologically internal and endosomatic forces makes it possible to retain some theoretical construct that accounts for the endogenous determinants of human behavior and experience, without having recourse to the somatic strategy. I will continue to use the term "drive" for this theoretical construct, although I do so hesitantly because of the conceptual (and political) baggage it carries. What tips the balance in favor of the term is based in clinical observation: I see that human life has a direction to it and a momentum behind it. There is an urgency to people's goals that gives their lives a special meaning. This urgency is not always (or even usually) conscious; a significant objective of analytic work is to help patients become more aware of how compelling their goals are, even when disavowed.

But the idea of drive looks very different once we have abandoned the somatic strategy. The most important difference is not thinking of drive as a stimulus. In contrast to the traditional view, I do not think of drive as a "something" that accumulates and requires discharge. The concept of

drive as I use it suggests a directedness that governs human behavior. Drive is a tendency, a characteristic of mind (even of human nature) that underlies all particular motives and through which stimuli acquire meaning. Thus, in line with Freud's view (especially the view embodied in his last dual-instinct theory), I see drive as an essential and irreducible element in all behavior and experience. The mind is exposed to any number of external stimuli, arising from the body and from the physical and interpersonal environments. Human experience is the result of these stimuli filtered through the psychological tendencies that I call the drives.

My approach, then, focuses analytic attention on the endogenous elements of behavior and experience without giving priority to bodily stimuli. I am left with certain questions—the same questions, actually, that Freud addressed in "Instincts and Their Vicissitudes." I will have to justify a theory based on a limited number of fundamental tendencies and to argue the utility of my particular choice of tendencies. For the moment, though, I will content myself with having demonstrated that Freud's particular dual-instinct theory is not biologically inevitable; its value must be fought out on psychological grounds alone.

Dualism Redux

FREUD'S vision of the passions that move us powered the development of psychoanalysis for many years. But an accumulating body of clinical evidence now suggests that what was once so liberating has become oppressive. Straining against the procrustean limits of the dual-instinct theory, many analysts have abandoned it. Some, broadly speaking those operating within the relational model of psychoanalysis, reject the idea of drive entirely. Others, hoping to preserve the original model by enlarging it, have grossly redefined the concept of drive or have added new drives to the system.

In Chapters 3 and 4 I argued that efforts to preserve libido and aggression at the theoretical core and attempts to get rid of drive entirely have weakened the interpretive power of psychoanalysis. Now I will try to show that this power can be saved by retaining *a* two-drive system, but *not* the libido/aggression theory.

Dualism is not particularly popular these days. Intellectually, it evokes visions of reductionism, a sense that one is precipitously, perhaps arrogantly, imposing order on a complex observational field. Clinically, advocating dualism provokes charges that one is retreating from the ineffable ambiguity of life itself. There is even a moral overtone to this charge: analysts force a patient's experience into a narrow framework to preserve their theoretical commitments. Thereby we sacrifice the patient's individuality on the altar of our own need to know. Edgar Levenson broadly criticizes "the attribution of purpose to behavior" because the idea of purpose itself "is defined by the therapist's hermeneutics—by what he thinks matters" (1972, p. 207).

Because of its unpopularity, I need to argue my preference for dualism

at the outset. I am inclined to say that dualism is to be preferred mainly because, like old age, it beats the alternative. More accurately, it beats the several alternatives that have been suggested: no-drive theories, one-drive theories, and multiple-drive theories.

Earlier I argued that attempts to get rid of drive entirely, if looked at carefully enough, inevitably contain theoretical constructs that serve the same conceptual functions as the drives. No-drive theories become one-drive theories. One-drive theories do not support a psychoanalytic vision of internal, pre-experiential conflict. So they do not support the presumption of personal agency, which rests on the idea that choices among various inner needs and desires determine how experience is organized and actions are pursued. One-drive theories cannot distinguish between inner conflict and frustration. Conflict is never simply personal; in one-drive theories it is always *with* the object. Theoretically, this quickly decays into a radical environmentalism; clinically it can lead to blaming the object (parent, spouse, boss, analyst) for the patient's unpleasant experiences.

For those analysts who have not sought to abandon drive entirely, the most popular theoretical option has been to increase the number of irreducible motivational forces. Thus Hartmann proposed the idea of noninstinctual energy, Jacobson introduced the concept of quantities of undifferentiated energy, and Mahler argued for an independent drive toward individuation. The major ego psychologists, each in his or her own way, quietly transformed psychoanalysis into a three-drive theory. This strategy has become the springboard for even more drastic revisionism among theorists who wish to maintain some ties with the ego-psychological framework.

Joseph Lichtenberg, for example, believes that there are five psychic motivational systems. Each "is built around a fundamental need, and each is based on behaviors clearly observable beginning in the neonatal period" (1988, p. 60; he has greatly elaborated this thesis in Lichtenberg, 1989). The motivational systems are irreducible, endogenous, and pre-experiential. They are, therefore, drives. Lichtenberg's five systems are: (1) the need to fulfill physiological requirements; (2) the need for attachment and affiliation; (3) the need for assertion and exploration; (4) the need to react aversively through antagonism or withdrawal; and (5) the need for sensual and sexual pleasure. More explicitly than most authors, Lichtenberg acknowledges his departure from the interpretive system of the dual-instinct theory: "in suggesting a sensual-sexual motivational-functional system as

one of five separate motivational-functional systems, I am in disagreement with many of the basic tenets of psychoanalysis" (1988, p. 69).

George Klein, in his ambitious revision of classical metapsychology, placed Freud's hedonistic sensibility at the center of his system: "My aim . . . is to reorient psychoanalytic theory to the essential wisdom of the pleasure principle—that we act so as to maximize pleasure or gratification and to minimize unpleasure of all kinds, especially anxiety" (1976, p. 213). But for Klein there are six distinguishable "vital" pleasures, which appear in infancy, become elaborated in the course of development, and are crucial in "the delineation of self-identity" (p. 217). These include: (1) pleasure in reduction of unpleasant tension; (2) sensual pleasure; (3) pleasure in functioning; (4) pleasure in experiencing the self as an effective agent of change—effectance pleasure; (5) pleasure in pleasing; and (6) pleasure in synthesis.

While Lichtenberg talks of "needs" and Klein of "pleasures," their models cover conceptually similar terrain. Both attempt to relieve the motivational system of the constraints imposed by Freud's dualism, and there is considerable overlap between the motives covered by Lichtenberg's five-drive and Klein's six-drive models. There is a similar sensibility in Daniel Stern's understanding of the motives that can be observed in neonates. He puts it this way:

> while there is no question that we need a concept of motivation, it clearly will have to be reconceptualized in terms of many discrete, but interrelated, motivational systems . . . [Further study] will be hampered if these motivational systems are assumed a priori to be derivatives of one or two basic, less definable instincts rather than more definable separate phenomena (1985, p. 238).

Stern attempts no comprehensive list of the motives he has defined. Instead he claims to have observed "a plethora of motivational systems that operate early, appear separable, and are backed by some imperative" (p. 238). He mentions among these motives: exploration; curiosity; perceptual preference; the search for cognitive novelty; pleasure in mastery; and attachment. There are certainly, he implies, many more.

Whereas some authors have suggested multiple-drive models, others have attempted to broaden the approach to motivation by mixing the sensibilities of different psychoanalytic models. Many analysts do this in their clinical work, drawing interpretations from their understanding of drive

theory or object relations theory or self psychology. Generally, model mixing remains private, perhaps even unformulated or not quite formulated by the analyst himself (Sandler, 1983), although sometimes the clinical implications of the strategy are spelled out (D. Silverman, 1986).

A variant of the model-mixing strategy that has been highly developed both theoretically and clinically appears in the work of Fred Pine. He writes:

> psychoanalytic theory, growing from clinical work, has found it useful to conceptualize the organization of experience around at least four features: drive development, ego function, internalized object relations, and, most recently, self organization and experience . . . no one of these four psychologies has absolute hierarchical superiority to any other. There *is* hierarchical organization in every individual, but this is a matter of personal history and not general theory (1985, p. 16).

Broadly speaking, Pine's drive-derived motives involve the attempt to satisfy wishes based in bodily urges and their vicissitudes in early familial relationships. Ego motives stem from defensive and adaptive needs dictated by the exigencies of external reality. Object-related motives are enactments of a childhood drama and represent attempts to assimilate novel, contemporary experience to a familiar template. Motives organized around self-experience represent attempts to maintain feelings of continuity, boundaries, and self-esteem (Pine 1985; 1988).

Each "psychology," as Pine describes it, represents a fundamental, irreducible motive system independent of the others. Each is an interpretive system; a scaffold on which a range of behaviors and experiences can be arrayed. Thus the four psychologies amount to four drives.

Pine brings these systems together in two different ways. Early in life, each system dominates experience at different moments in the day: at different times the child pursues drive-derived needs, is preoccupied with the exercise of ego functions, is primarily involved with its objects, or is most concerned with its own evolving self (1985, p. 22). Thus, for example, "The child in the anal phase is not living an all-anal life" (p. 40), and "the normal symbiotic phase . . . is not 'all symbiosis' for the infant" (p. 41). Later on, experience is more complex in its determination, and the principle of multiple function guarantees that the demands of each system will be taken into account at all times:

> Just as an emphasis on moments of experience, varying in their prime content, impact, and subsequent organization, permits reconciliation of the

competing demands of drive, ego, and object relations theories upon the child's developmental time, so the concept of multiple function permits integration of the place of these theoretical points of view in the developmental actualities of the child's life—that is, they become integrated in the person, whatever theory has to say (p. 65).

Multiple-drive and mixed-model approaches have become increasingly popular as disenchantment with classical dualism has spread. They embody an apparent openness to the wide range of human experience and a reasonable, broad-minded analytic attitude. Nevertheless, I believe that they are weak where theory is needed most, in facilitating the clinical goals of psychoanalytic inquiry. To demonstrate this, I will spell out, highly schematically, five steps in the construction and communication of an analytic interpretation:

1. The patient talks about whatever she wants to talk about. The content of her associations may or may not reflect any special psychological awareness. That is, the thoughts may be introspective—reports of fantasies, desires, beliefs, and so on—or they may be more commonplace, conversational, and unreflective. Sometimes the patient is not talking at all, since silence (whether thoughtful, fearful, depressive, or angry and withholding) and other nonverbal enactments have their place in free association.

2. The analyst listens and observes. There is a great deal to observe within the psychoanalytic situation: words, tone, physical presence, affective ambience, countertransference reactions, and so on. The analyst is constantly deciding where to direct her attention. Trains of thought lead off in all directions. The analyst must think about which are most profitably pursued at any moment and which can be left for later. "Free-floating attention" requires a great deal of activity, not all of it conscious.

3. On the basis of this activity, the analyst imposes a framework on the observational field. This framework not only determines how the data of the analysis will be interpreted, but which of the virtually limitless number of events will be considered data in the first place. Does the patient's new haircut have special significance today? What about her relatively less precise use of words? Should the analyst immerse herself in persistent thoughts about her own upcoming vacation, or should this be overcome as an unwarranted distraction?

4. The framework that the analyst imposes on the data illuminates an aspect of the patient's experience, or a perspective on it, that was previously hidden. This newly illuminated idea becomes the nucleus of an interpretation. The idea itself may derive primarily from a new way of

understanding the patient's words (the cigar she's talking about is a penis); it may be a way of understanding her actions (the silence is an angry provocation); it may reflect the analyst's assessment of her own countertransference (her preoccupation with vacation is an identification with the patient's self-absorbed father and recreates the patient's experience of abandonment).

5. The analyst formulates her impressions in a relatively economical way and communicates them to the patient. When this works, the interpretation stays reasonably close to the patient's experience, but not too close. It is not only in the connection but also in the discrepancy between the patient's experience and the analyst's interpretation that the gap between the unconscious and consciousness gets bridged.

Understanding the interpretive process in terms of these five steps illuminates an important relationship between the analyst's theory and the clinical process: Making the unconscious conscious depends partly on the analyst's empathy, but also on her having a perspective that is different from the patient's. If she did not, step 4 could not take place; the analyst would be bound by the patient's conscious experience. The cigar would be a cigar, the silence just a break in the flow of thoughts, the intrusive concern with vacation just a piece of laziness. Clinical psychoanalysis depends on the analyst's own narrative structure (Spence, 1982), her storyline (Schafer, 1983), or what Freud called the ability to provide the patient with "conscious anticipatory ideas" (1909).

Let me illustrate this point with an example of Roy Schafer's. He is using some clinical material to demonstrate the theoretical weaknesses of a biologically based energy model for psychoanalysis. But at the same time, he remains a strong proponent of an interpretive system that assumes the motivational primacy of sexual and aggressive wishes. Schafer describes

> a certain patient's struggle against homosexual transference. That struggle frequently took the form of his promptly forgetting major developments in his analytic hours. Upon analysis, it seemed that: this forgetting defended against his getting more deeply involved in his analysis since that involvement would lead into experiencing and disclosing the homosexual transference; it represented him as a woman with a vagina, i.e., suitable as a homosexual object; and the forgetting was intended to provoke attacks by the analyst, thus bringing about repetitions of sadomasochistically colored attacks by his father, and thereby amounted to an unconscious homosexual seduction (1976, p. 85).

It took some excellent analytic work to arrive at the conclusions Schafer describes. Armed with his interpretive perspective, he will be in a good position to do the sort of "making the unconscious conscious" that expands patients' experience of themselves and their circumstances. Schafer will, as a result of this work, be able to give poignant meaning to what the patient probably had thought was simply an unpleasant, unexpected intrusion into his relationship with the analyst. By providing a motivational (and life-historical) context, this will significantly broaden the patient's appreciation of himself and will facilitate similar searches after deepened meaning in the future.

But the effectiveness of Schafer's work, I suggest, depends on his having a limited vision of what was happening with the patient—a vision that, unlike Pine's, does not assume that the meaning of experience changes from moment to moment or that it expresses a wide range of motives. Let us return to the beginning of the vignette and consider the data that need to be explained. The only datum Schafer presents is that this patient frequently forgets aspects of his sessions. Even the idea that what he has forgotten are "major developments" is an interpretation imposed on the data. They are major from the analyst's point of view; the patient may or may not agree.

Certainly the various functions—defenses, identifications, covert gratifications—attributed to the forgetting are interpretations. Presumably they have been arrived at jointly, but certainly they have been significantly influenced by the analyst's preconceptions. And the idea that the warded-off transference is best characterized as homosexual is without question a theory of the analyst's. (We don't know, and it is ultimately irrelevant, whether it is also a theory of the patient's.)

Analysts working with other interpretive systems would find other explanations for the patient's forgetting. They would even explain why the patient had sexualized the act of forgetting. I am not suggesting that these alternatives are better or more powerful, but I do want to mention a few possibilities. For one, the transference could involve not fear of homosexuality, but fear of loss of self. Or it could be organized around guilt and fear over having abandoned a parent in favor of a new relationship with the analyst. Perhaps the patient feels anxious about being competent enough to remember, so that forgetting is a way of making the analyst feel useful.

Any of these formulations might, with a particular patient at a particular time, serve the goals of analysis. But the formulation is not the event, and

it is not even the patient's experience of the event as it is happening. The homosexual transference that Schafer interpreted, though I believe it a powerful tool for promoting analytic goals, is not a fact but a construction drawn from his theory.

Where do multiple-drive or mixed-model theories leave us? In Pine's terms, the patient's silence might represent a drive-derived need (along the lines Schafer suggests). But it might also embody an ego solution (to the conflict posed by the patient's commitment to analysis on the one hand and his desire for privacy on the other). Perhaps it does enact a noninstinctually driven object relationship (it recreates the uncomfortable experience of being with a withdrawn, depressed mother, and the analyst's very urge to interpret it as a resistance is a sign of his countertransferential identification with the neglected child). Or it could reflect the patient's evolving sense of self-cohesion (because it is a statement of autonomy through defiance of the analyst's values or of the treatment itself). What theoretical guide do we have that might lead us to prefer one interpretation to any other?

Pine most likely would answer that we know by listening to the patient, that the patient's own associations will be our guide. But this raises two problems. First, once we accept a multiple-drive or mixed-model framework, who is to say how many drives (or, in Pine's terms, psychologies) are to be included in the system? Pine says there are four. Lichtenberg suggests five. Klein finds six. Stern acknowledges "a plethora." Theoretically there is no reason to stop at any particular place. Clinically, if the analyst does not feel comfortable interpreting a particular thought as deriving from some other, disavowed thought, he can simply posit a new, irreducible drive. For example, if the analyst recoils from confronting the patient (or himself) with the possibility that the patient's ambitions represent aim-inhibited homicidal attacks on his father, he can invoke a drive to mastery that avoids any need to address aggression. Although any theory can be used to rationalize the analyst's avoidance, this is a special problem for open-ended models.

Perhaps more important, multiple-drive and mixed-model theories put the analyst in the position of listening with what is essentially a kind of naive atheoretical or pretheoretical empathy. Theory supplies the guidelines—the basic rules of procedure—to support the idea that one mental content is inevitably a transformation of some other mental content. Without these, the interpretation never gets beyond what the patient is saying. The interpreting analyst needs some construct that gives warrant for as-

suming that the patient's experience is more than it seems to be. There must be something in our theory that allows us to interpret reported fantasies of self-fragmentation as reflecting fears of losing connections to an object, or castration fears as derivatives of concerns about the integrity of the self. But this also means that the analyst's interpretive system cannot be infinitely expandable. Multiple-drive and mixed-model theories do not support the analyst's having a perspective that is not the patient's. Without an alternative perspective, a cigar *is* just a cigar, at least so long as the patient says it is.

This is a special problem when the patient is in a resistant frame of mind—when he insists, for example, that the he has simply run out of things to say or when he admits under duress that the silence is a failure of imagination. Why don't we just accept this at face value? Why are we sure that the silence is a not-wanting-to-speak (or a not-wanting-to-know or a not-wanting-to relate)? Our conviction that the silence is motivated at all is theoretically based. But without this conviction, we could not facilitate our patients' expanded recognition of their own experience. The patient's awareness of a dynamic unconscious—*the very existence of a dynamic unconscious in an experientially vital form*—depends upon the analyst's having some conceptual tool that links the spoken with the unspoken, and eventually with the unspeakable. The analyst must be able to focus on the derivation of available thoughts from unavailable but more fundamental ones. From the beginning, providing this conceptual tool has been the clinical role of drive.

The conclusion, admittedly, is uncomfortable. Dualism (Schafer's or anyone else's) is limiting, and it has been a problem from the very beginnings of psychoanalytic inquiry. Consider everything that Freud overlooked about Dora. For thirty years at least there has been a thriving cottage industry devoted to detailing what Freud should have discovered, but didn't, in this three-month fragment of an analysis. But the same constraints that limit dualistic frameworks also make them penetrating; they make it possible to arrive at those unexpected, often unwelcome reworkings of experience that we consider the contents of the dynamic unconscious.

The situation is similar to what Peter Gay describes in his discussion of how historians construct history. Gay first acknowledges the conventional view that a broad perspective, an open-mindedness, should lead to factual accuracy. Accordingly, personal idiosyncrasies must interfere with clarity, warping the historian's vision: "The historian's style . . . is a repository of

biases and his perception of causes is bound to be compromised by . . . crippling ideological burdens." This compromised perception parallels the distortions caused by the analyst's commitment to a narrow interpretive system. But, Gay continues, things are not so simple: "style can also be a privileged passage to historical knowledge and . . . the historian's particular vision of what made the past world move, however distorted that vision may be by his neuroses, professional deformations, or class prejudices, may yet assist him in securing insights into his material that he could not have gained without them" (1985, pp. viii–ix). The narrow instrument is also sharp; it penetrates beneath the surface.

I would make a similar claim for a dualistic motivational system. Freud missed a great deal about Dora, and his attempt at analysis was a therapeutic failure. But the work illuminated a dimension of human experience that could never have been revealed without an overriding commitment to the libido theory. Joseph Smith is being extravagant when he calls Freud's drive theory the idea that changed the world, but he has caught the power that comes with a narrow interpretive vision.

It is not only the narrowness of dualism that empowers it. More important, human experience is indelibly marked with the radical polarities that are most poignant at the very beginning of life. For the infant, things are good or bad, and they are present or absent. The pleasure and the reality principles respectively address these unbridgeable alternatives and the way they continue to govern the mind forever. Smith puts it this way: "the interval between wish (absence of the object) and satisfaction (presence of the object) [is where] it all begins—desire, rage, imaging, thinking, language, object relations, and structural development" (1986, p. 563).

With development, dichotomies fade and nuances dominate. It is generally considered a sign of maturity when either/or gives way to both/and. Within the terms of Freud's drive theory, this progression is explained by concepts like sublimation, neutralization, aim inhibition, instinctual fusion, and the like—all of them developmental achievements. But, each in its own way, they are also farfetched and problematic (see Schafer, 1976, for an especially incisive critique). So there is a temptation for theorists to be mature in their theorizing, to avoid the "childish" lure of dualistic oversimplification.

I think, however, that in rejecting dualism we lose our sense of the dilemma of "yes or no" as it shapes the origin of experience and of life itself. And we lose the persistence of polarity in the organization even of

adult experience. I agree with Smith, who concludes that he cannot "quickly dismiss the idea that life is organized around and in terms of great polarities like presence-absence, danger-defense, pathologically narcissistic-object related, progression-regression, life-death" (1986, p. 566).

A New Dualism

Thoughts about the power of dualism and the narrowness of Freud's drive model have led me to consider possible alternatives to the libido/aggression theory. I begin with the idea of "feeling states," a concept borrowed from the work of Joseph Sandler. Feeling states, which may be conscious or unconscious, are multiply determined experiences, shaped by both internal and external events (Joffe and Sandler, 1968). The internal events involve the ebb and flow of a wide range of physiological and psychological needs, and they are affected by the state of the body generally. The external events refer to conditions in the person's immediate interpersonal world, as well as in the larger environment.

Feeling states are organizers of the drives; they are the experiential indicators of how well the drive needs are being met. The quality of a person's feeling state at any time reflects an assessment of personal circumstances; in doing so, they guide action. An important determinant of feeling states is the status (actual, anticipated, and potential satisfactions or frustrations) of motives.* They are like highway signs, conveying information about where we are and perhaps about where we will get if we continue along the same route. But they don't say anything about where we *want* to go and they don't provide the energy to get us there. This is where the drives themselves enter the theoretical picture: we can think of drives as aiming at the creation of specific feeling states.

I believe there are two quite different feeling states that can usefully be thought of as the aims of fundamental drives. One is the sense of physical and emotional well-being—freedom from the pressure of any urgent need and the absence of unpleasant affects of which anxiety is the prototype. There is a conviction that one can relax, that it is all right to surrender,

---

*Here I am departing considerably from Sandler, who believes that feeling states themselves are motives (1972, p. 296). Sandler's uneconomical formulation reflects his attempt to preserve the libido/aggression theory. Feeling states become a parallel but separate motivational system, existing alongside the drives and intertwined with them in confusing and frequently implausible ways.

actively, to circumstances. There is a sense of continuity that verges on timelessness; neither the well-being nor the conditions that produce it will ever change. I call the search for this feeling state the "safety drive."

The second feeling state, in contrast, involves the sense of vitality and vigorousness; the experience is of being alive and active. It is the feeling that Mahler caught so accurately and poignantly in her description of the child's exuberance during the practicing subphase of separation-individuation (1968). We see it in the athlete who has just won a race, arms raised and head tilted back, feeling the fullest sense of self. And we each experience it in our everyday lives when we have achieved a goal, overcome an obstacle, felt that we have used ourselves well. It is a feeling of being effective, stimulated, perhaps excited. In contrast to the timelessness of the first feeling state, time seems to fly by. The underlying conviction is not that circumstances will stay the same but that they will change, and change for the better. I will use a term coined by Robert White (1959, 1963) and call the search for this feeling state the "effectance drive."

Like any dualism—any attempt at classification, really—the one I'm proposing is somewhat arbitrary; both the feeling states and the drives could be organized differently. But each of the drives has a long history in psychoanalytic theorizing; their importance has been recognized by analysts beginning with Freud. More important, the decision to base a theoretical formulation on safety and effectance needs is based on their power to explain how clinical psychoanalysis works. Patients come to analysis in the first place because they feel thwarted in doing what they want to do or believe they can do (in work, in love, in experiencing a particular quality of life). Once analysis gets under way, we are constantly attuned to the tension between progressive phases (involving risk taking, trying new acts and new thoughts) and fearful retreats from risk. Analysis works in the gap between perceived security and perceived novelty. I believe, then, that as analysts we are immersed constantly in our patients' conflicting needs for safety and effectiveness. Summarizing the relationship between the treatment setting and patients' ability to work analytically, Pine has written that the atmosphere of "noncondemnation, reality orientation, survival, and positive valuation [of the patient, by the analyst]—provide a *context of safety* in which growth can take place . . . and in which ventures toward change can be risked" (1985, p. 171).

Pine's comment conveys a sense that the patient experiences analysis as a dialectic between the risk of trying out new possibilities and the safety of the familiar. It is surprising that this experience has not been integrated

into the motivational theory of psychoanalysis. Freud based his drive model on a clinical phenomenon: he argued that transference, and especially the erotic transference, stood as the best proof of the libido theory. I suggest that we are entitled to revise the drive theory in light of our own clinical findings.

The safety and effectance drives share certain conceptual characteristics with libido and aggression. They are endogenous and pre-experiential; from the beginning of life they have a direction, which is innate. Because of this they give shape to all experience. Their expression—the particular motives to which they give rise—are decisively influenced by interpersonal events, but the underlying tendencies are immutable. Because of this, the behaviors motivated by the drives are enormously variable. All behaviors satisfy some of the requirements of each drive. The safety and effectance needs themselves are generally not experienced directly or consciously, although they will be in some circumstances.

Like libido and aggression in Freud's model, the safety and effectance drives are conceptually irreducible—they cannot be broken down into simpler psychological units. Because of this, they are separate from each other, and there is an inherent tension between them. The strength of each drive varies from person to person. Some people value safety and security above all else; others are constantly seeking stimulation and even risk. This variation is constitutional and is probably a significant aspect of temperamental differences in children.

The Safety Drive

The unique psychotherapy that Freud called analysis began with a disquieting observation: people who are significantly disabled by their symptoms and who believe they want help nevertheless have great difficulty following a simple procedure that offers the possibility of relief. The patients are told that improvement depends upon their willingness to speak freely about whatever comes to mind. That is all, the rest is in the analyst's hands. But the simple rule turns out to be nearly impossible to follow, no matter how consciously devoted to the process the patient is.

It took Freud many years of technical experimentation to come up with a method that addressed patients' fears or their reticence or their defiance. But the difficulty in following the free-association rule remains, with every patient, throughout every analysis. Resistance is a fact of life for each of us, beginning with its appearance in our own training analyses. In a sense,

with every new patient, it is always a surprise and always feels like an unwelcome intrusion. This is true even long after we have accepted it intellectually as an inevitable and essential part of treatment.

The endless, always disturbing encounters with resistance teach a powerful lesson: people do not and cannot speak freely until something happens to convince them that it is prudent to do so. Even if they believe that it is useful to speak freely, they will not until they feel safe enough. Freud himself addressed the problem of safety, theoretically, when he revised his views on anxiety in 1926. The central element of his new formulation was the idea that the expression of a drive-derived impulse—any impulse, no matter how powerful, urgent, or potentially pleasurable—will be curbed if the person senses that expressing the impulse will be dangerous. This clearly implies that feeling safe is a motive even stronger than pleasure seeking itself (Sandler and Joffe, 1968; Ogden, 1989).

Over the years, an ever-increasing number of authors have pointed out that the patient's feelings of safety are crucial to progress in analysis. Strikingly, this emphasis has come from analysts of all theoretical persuasions; it seems to emerge independently of any preconceptions. In his seminal paper on psychoanalytic technique, Strachey (1934) wrote that free association becomes possible only when patients can experience the benign presence of the analyst. The analyst becomes an "auxiliary superego" for the patient, a new object less prone to criticize and condemn. In a similar vein, but in terms not influenced by metapsychological necessity, Sullivan suggested that treatment really gets under way when "the patient begins to feel safe in saying various things to the interviewer which ordinarily he would not say" (1954, p. 231).

More recently, Roy Schafer (1983) has written of the need to establish an "atmosphere of safety" in the analysis and traces this prescription back to Freud's technical papers. Weiss, Sampson, and their colleagues (1986) present impressive empirical evidence that analysis progresses when patients feel safe enough to risk thinking and saying new kinds of things about themselves. Fred Pine has written beautifully about the kinds of interventions that promote feelings of safety, as has Paul Myerson (1981a, b). Both believe that, for many patients at least, providing a safe context occupies "center stage in therapeutic work" (Pine, 1985, p. 133).

These formulations suggest that people will not risk either new kinds of behavior or awareness of new kinds of experience unless they feel safe enough to do so. Progressive change, even mental health itself, will be sacrificed because of perceived feelings of danger. This convergence of

clinical judgment is particularly striking because it comes as a surprise; it flies in the face of technical prescriptions organized around the need to frustrate the patient's desire and to enforce a rule of abstinence. Schafer's creative reading of Freud to the contrary, each of the authors I have mentioned, and many more who stress the importance of creating an atmosphere of safety, has turned his back on established technical teaching. Each has done so because of what he has learned in the course of doing the actual work of psychoanalysis. It is no overstatement to assert that the importance of feelings of safety is one of the strongest findings that has emerged from a century of psychoanalytic investigation.

Despite the force of this finding, safety has largely remained a theoretical loose end. Neither Freud nor others who shared his commitment to dualism and his reluctance to abandon the libido/aggression theory have found a place for safety in the drive model. Sandler, although he denies that the need to feel safe is a drive (1962), writes that it is "the dominant criterion in determining the activity of the psychic apparatus" (Sandler and Joffe, 1969, p. 245). Consider the similarity of this formulation to Freud's assertion that drive is "the ultimate cause of all activity" (1940, p. 148). The failure of Sandler and others to see that, in the terms of their own clinical sensibility, they have made safety a drive is due to a partisan but conceptually vestigial loyalty to an abandoned model.

THE WORKINGS of the safety drive invariably move people closer to their objects. This idea has roots going back to the early history of psychoanalysis. Not long after he introduced the drive model, Freud addressed the origin of our attachment to objects. The first connection between infant and mother, he said, is not explained by libidinal needs; rather, it serves the ego instincts. Unlike the sexual instincts, which can be satisfied autoerotically from the start and then through fantasy, the ego instincts require an external object from the very beginning. The infant's pleasure needs permit a delay in object choice and support wide latitude in the object that is ultimately selected. In contrast, the self-preservative needs bring the infant immediately and specifically to the mother. "Ego-strivings," Freud wrote in his unpublished "Overview of the Transference Neuroses," "from the beginning are directed at object[s]" (1987, p. 11).

This comment underscores an important feature of the ego instincts: in contrast to the sexual drives, the object of the ego instincts is necessarily another person. The infant can survive, Freud tells us, because it is cared for by a mother (1911a, p. 220n). In this respect the ego instincts operate

similarly to the safety drive, which is inherently and from the beginning directed at a human object. (Early in life this object is a figure in reality, but in the course of development safety needs are directed toward internalized objects as well.) I believe this recaptures some of the wisdom of Freud's first dual-instinct theory that was lost when he eliminated the ego instincts from the system and replaced them with libido and aggression, neither of which supports an innate connection to the world of other people.

The Effectance Drive

Like the safety drive, the effectance drive has a long history in psychoanalytic thinking. Analysts, and other psychologists as well, have repeatedly observed the pleasure that everybody takes in acquiring and exercising new capabilities. Erikson, for example, describes how "a child who has just found himself able to walk . . . seems driven to repeat the act for the pure delight of functioning, and out of the need to master and perfect a newly initiated function" (1963, p. 235).

The need that drives the child's urgent, exuberant activity has been given different names by different observers. While they differ in nuance and in some of their implications, each represents an attempt to describe what Hendrick has succinctly called the need "to do and to learn how to do" (1942, p. 40). This has been variously referred to as: joy in being a cause (Groos, 1901); pleasure in functioning *(Funktionlust)* (Bühler, 1918); the instinct to master (Hendrick, 1942, 1943); the push toward ego synthesis (Erikson, 1963); the urge to motility (Mittelman, 1954); effectance motivation (White, 1959, 1963); and the drive toward individuation (Mahler, Pine, and Bergman, 1975). It is the need reflected in recent interpretations of the concept of ego instincts, by Plaut (1984) and Stern (1985).

Unfortunately, the effectance drive has been a major bone of contention since psychoanalysis became polarized by its first major defection. Alfred Adler's insistence on a primary drive for power or mastery precipitated his break with Freud (Anspacher and Anspacher, 1956). Although even earlier (in response to Groos) Freud had considered and rejected a power drive (1905c), after Adler's defection the issue acquired a special poignancy. In "On the History of the Psycho-Analytic Movement" Freud was particularly emphatic, even vitriolic, about the idea. Adler's emphasis on

self-assertion and power, he claimed, represent "the twisted interpretations and distortions of the disagreeable facts of analysis" (1914b, p. 54).

By taking this harsh stance, Freud made it difficult for his followers to integrate their observations about the importance of effectance needs into the motivational system of psychoanalysis. A number of authors have gotten around the problem by attributing these needs to the ego rather than to the drives. Thus Erikson presented the need for synthesis as a characteristic of the ego (1963), and Winnicott went so far as to trace the very origins of the ego to the infant's experience of omnipotence (1962). Sandler described pleasures based in ego functions that operate independently of sexual and aggressive impulses (Sandler and Joffe, 1965, 1966).

What this strategy does, of course, is to create parallel and independent motivational systems that resist integration and frustrate attempts at theoretical synthesis. Rapaport took this approach to an extreme—and inadvertently demonstrated its bankruptcy—in his distinction between motives and causes (1960). He managed to define motives so narrowly (especially in terms of the buildup and discharge of tensions) that only Freud's viscerogenic drives qualify. Other goal-directed activity—explicitly including White's effectance-driven activities—are not motivated at all, but merely "caused" (p. 854).

When we have separated drive from ego motives, we can no longer integrate different motivational tendencies. The effect is even more powerful when we distinguish motives from causes, implying that the two classes of intention operate in discrete universes of discourse. The whole purpose of Freud's drive theory—the hierarchical arrangement of fundamental and derivative motives—is defeated.

Some authors have attempted to blend effectance into the classical drive theory. This usually takes the form of introducing a third drive. Hendrick, for example, suggests that there is a fundamental "instinct to master" which aims toward "the pleasure in executing a function successfully, regardless of its sensual value" (1942, p. 41). The workings of this drive can be observed in "the need to learn how to do things, manifested in the infant's practice of its sensory, motor, and intellectual means for mastering its environment" (p. 34). The urgency of this practicing can be seen in the child's absorption, often at a level that seems compulsive, in repeating a new activity until it is comfortably mastered.

White, like Hendrick, based his concept of effectance on the observation of children's play and exploration. He was impressed by children's push

toward using physical, cognitive, and psychological capacities as they develop, and by their pride in accomplishment and pleasure in mastering the demands of reality. Effectance motives operate continuously and reflect a tendency guiding all activity. The satisfaction that accompanies effectance is "a feeling of efficacy," connected to the child's sense of competence at altering reality in one way or another (p. 35). The force behind effectance motives, White says, is derived from "independent ego energies." Effectance "is a gentle motive without compulsive pressure" (1963, p. 147), but it is still "as basic as anything in human nature" (p. 24).

THERE is a clear consensus in the sensibilities of all these authors. Although Hendrick refers to a drive, White to an independent ego energy, Sandler and Erikson to ego functions, and Rapaport to causes as distinct from motives, each agrees that there is a class of activities guided by the need to feel that one is doing what one can do, using one's capacities fully and effectively. The child's urgent striving to do what she has never done before, her exuberance when she achieves her goal, and her joyous repetition of newly acquired capacities reflect a fundamental characteristic of human nature. Children's play, exploration, and intellectual curiosity, all point in the same direction.

These activities do not end with the passing of childhood. Grownups play games, they travel, they create art and ideas, and they jump out of airplanes with parachutes. Each of these activities expresses an irresistible imperative of human life: we must do what can be done, and we must do it as well as possible. This constitutes a drive in any psychologically meaningful sense of the term.

The effectance drive, like the safety drive, aims at producing a particular internal feeling state. While I agree with White and others that feeling able to affect reality is an important part of the experience I am describing, my emphasis is much more on an inner sensation. It is a sensation that begins in the body, probably in the muscles, and is initially experienced as pleasure in movement for movement's sake alone. Soon after, it expands to include the early sense of agency that Stern (1985) believes the infant feels when he first experiences volitional acts, such as deliberate movement. Later in the course of development it is extended outward, becoming inextricably involved with feelings of competence and mastery over the environment.

I have suggested that because it aims at feelings of physical, intellectual, and psychological relaxation, the safety drive moves us closer to other

people. In contrast, the feeling state that is the aim of effectance is characterized by a sense of self-sufficiency, autonomy, and individuation. White has put it this way: "Effectance, leading as it does to increased competence in dealing with the environment, can be conceived of as inherently an urge away from the necessity for being mothered" (1963, p. 77).

The effectance drive is, therefore, a construct well suited to account for what are, unquestionably, aversive elements inherent in all object relations. Freud used aggression (and even the death instinct) to explain wishes to move away from the object. The hypothesis of an effectance drive fills a major gap in psychoanalytic object relations theory: how to explain antagonism that is neither a reaction to the object's failure nor the derivative of a primary, endogenous destructiveness.

Conflict Intrapsychic and Interpersonal

I believe that a dualistic drive theory organized around safety and effectance motives supports the psychoanalytic vision of human conflict even more fully than does Freud's libido/aggression model. I will discuss conflict within the terms of my hypothesis under three headings: conflict between opposing feeling states that is pre-experiential and may have little or no connection with other people; conflict about the object that precedes relatedness itself and contributes to the characteristics of whatever relationship is established; and conflict with the object, or interpersonal conflict.

The feeling states that are the aim of the safety and effectance drives differ in two important respects, regardless of the interpersonal situation within which they occur. The first differences involve the levels of tension or stimulation that are experienced physically, intellectually, and emotionally. We are all aware of how good it can feel sometimes to be stimulated, alert, vigorous, and energetic. But at other times these same feelings are stressful and exhausting. Then we will crave a release from the tension, even a surrender of our vitality. Effectance motives lead us to pursue heightened feelings; athletes even welcome pain, not because they are masochistic but because the pain is a sign that they are effectively pushing their bodies to a limit. In contrast, the safety drive aims at a feeling state that is more or less anaesthetic; we want to empty ourselves of feelings, even feelings that are often pleasurable.

The second difference involves the dissimilar sense of time characterizing the two feeling states. The safety drive aims at a feeling of continuity,

changelessness, even timelessness itself. Relaxing and releasing tension brings with it a renunciation of any concerns about a future. To the extent that a person feels safe, he believes that he will always feel safe, and this means that nothing will happen. In stark contrast, effectance aims at a feeling state in which something is happening, has happened, and will continue to happen. The future, progress, and change are essential. The same sense of timelessness that makes feeling safe so gratifying would stifle effectance needs.

Although I could be describing a temporal sequence in which one set of aims gives way to another, things are not so simple. The safety and effectance drives operate continuously and *both* pulls are *always* present, although one or another is likely to dominate conscious experience at any particular moment. Freud said that there is something in the nature of the sexual drive itself that precludes its full satisfaction (1912b, 1930). By suggesting two drives that move us in irreconcilably opposite directions, I am trying to capture some of his sense of the inexorable ambivalence of human life. This ambivalence, and the motivational conflicts to which it gives rise, are fundamental to human nature and can be considered independently of any object relations in which they get expressed.

THE SECOND type of conflict that develops out of the differences between safety and effectance motives is conflict *about* the object. I have already suggested that our safety needs push us toward other people while effectance needs pull us away. This suggests one way of understanding the often described tension between merger wishes (in the sense of life-long tendencies to surrender functional capacities to the object) and the desires to separate and individuate. From the beginning, the aim of the effectance drive is to own, use, feel, and master one's own body. Effectance drives the individuation process. In sharp contrast, the workings of the safety drive can lead us to give ourselves over to another person in the hope that our tensions will disappear through their ministrations. We are constantly moved to renounce not only competence, but autonomy itself.

Addressing this issue in Freud's terms, Peter Gay has written that culture is "indispensable and stifling at the same time." We might, all of us, be stifled (I think Gay means that we would surrender our individuality entirely) were it not for our drives. "What may rescue the individual from [culture's] fatal embrace are his instinctual urges; Freud's insistence on the drives' unremitting search for pleasure, which is anchored in his essential endowment" (1985, p. 175).

I would revise Gay's formulation. Culture, as a broad reverberation of human needs for relatedness, is indispensable because it serves our need for safety, for being embedded in a secure structure (Fromm, 1941). But it is stifling because it can thwart effectance strivings, which often push against the norms of social living. The same ambivalence that characterizes our most intimate object relations also colors our relationship to society at large.

Finally, we come to conflict with the object. I have argued in Chapter 4 that this is the only sort of conflict that can be explained by one-drive theories. In Freud's dualistic theory, however, conflict with the object is subordinated to the other two sources of conflict. I don't believe that this is inherent in dualism; rather, it derives from the theoretical position of sexuality in Freud's system.

From nearly the beginning (1896, p. 167n) to the very end (1940, p. 186) of his career, Freud saw sexuality as the only instigator of conflict. The problem with this is that sexuality is just the sort of need that directs our attention toward conflicts between the individual and "society"—*any* society. Consider the way George Klein understands conflict: "the require-ment for [sexual] control itself remains invariant [in all societies]; it is secured by the universal incest taboo and by the necessity for guiding and insuring the joining of sensuality to appropriate heterosexual expression" (1976, p. 91). Klein reached the following conclusion:

> A mother gratifies in all sorts of ways, but beyond a certain age one must not acknowledge her as a specific source of sensual experience. Other pleasures, as for instance . . . "effectance" pleasure, are probably never subject to so severe a rule of severance (p. 90).

I believe that this misrepresents what happens in families, and that when applied clinically it can be dangerously misleading. If we are not bound by the constraints inherent in Klein's theoretical commitment, we can notice that particular mothers (and of course particular fathers as well) require the renunciation of all sorts of capacities and their associated pleasures as the price for continued intimacy. Some require that the child renounce sensual demands, others that he give up aggression, adventurousness, competitiveness, independent judgment, high-intensity affect, idealizing tendencies, reality testing, and so on.

The list is endless, but the phenomenon has been described by theorists from Sullivan (who believed that the range of permissible motives was limited by parental anxiety) to Stern (who emphasized the ebbs and flows

of parental attunement to a range of affective and motivational states). These formulations all imply that (in my terms) any move toward effectance can embroil the child in conflict with others. I would add that safety needs can do the same. Because they propel the child toward the parent, they expose the child to the parent's feelings about being approached or needed or intruded upon. Safety needs can also involve the child, dangerously, in conflicts between his parents. Consider what happens when one parent feels jealous or wounded because the child has approached the other parent for comfort at a moment of crisis. The child can come to feel that his approach (even his preference at certain times for one parent) has alienated him from the other parent.

Klein missed this precisely because the *average expectable* environment is more obviously opposed to expressions of unbridled sexuality than it would be to expressions of unbridled effectance or safety needs. The average expectable environment can be presumed to oppose uninhibited sexual activity, which would be a threat both to family structure and to the gene pool. From this, many analysts conclude that all interpersonal conflict can be derived from the broad requirement to restrict sexual or aggressive expression. The revised drive theory focuses on particular rather than average expectable environments. Thus it lends itself to a more microscopic, critical examination of the interpersonal context within which conflict arises. By starting with safety and effectance drives, we can do more than account for pre-experiential conflict; we have a powerful framework for conceptualizing experientially induced (interpersonal) conflict as well.

I WILL conclude this chapter with some comments on something I believe has had a seriously detrimental impact on psychoanalytic theory and clinical work: Heinz Hartmann's idea of "autonomous" ego functions and the "conflict-free sphere" to which they give rise (1939a). Erikson (1962) neatly characterized the conflict-free sphere as a "miserly" concept; it drains vitality from psychoanalytic understanding. Yet Hartmann recognized that psychoanalysis needed such a concept, because of the narrowness of its drive theory. Many mental functions, he saw, operate outside the influence of libidinal or aggressive determinants. But because only libido and aggression can by definition become embroiled in conflict, these other functions must be conflict-free.

The problem with Hartmann's reasoning is that it does not stand up to clinical experience. For example, Weiss, Sampson, and their colleagues

write, "A young boy may . . . come to believe that almost any impulse, attitude, or goal is dangerous in that he would, by expressing the impulse or attitude or by pursuing the goal, risk the disruption of his ties to a parent and thus leave himself insufficiently protected or cared for" (1986, pp. 7–8). Accordingly, any motive can be the source of conflict. Stern addresses the theoretical issue this way: "Because it is no longer reasonable to think in terms of the general drives of eros and thanatos . . . the 'autonomous' in autonomous ego function has lost much of its meaning" (1985, p. 239).

I would take it even further. Every motive and every function are potentially (perhaps even inevitably) a source of conflict. We do not move forward without relinquishing something valued. We do not take care of ourselves without leaving behind some measure of our gratifying dependence on others, and we do not ask for or accept caretaking without yielding part of our own capability. There is no victory without some measure of loss.

It is the task of clinical analysis to reveal the conflicts that infiltrate every facet of our patients' lives, especially when they frustrate growth. The conflict-free sphere severely limits our power because it dictates that where there is conflict there must also be disclaimed lust or hatred. The modified dualism I propose, with its support for an expanded vision of pre-experiential conflict, conflict about the object, and conflict with the object, will enrich our capacity to engage the wide range of dilemmas that are inherent in living.

Structural Concepts

Clinical Interpretation and Psychic Structure

MODELS of the mind are maps. Like all maps, they are made to serve a particular purpose and are drawn on the basis of certain assumptions. Although these assumptions are highly abstract and even arcane, the usefulness of the maps lies in their ability to help us do something quite concrete—to get from one place to another. The same can certainly be said of psychoanalytic theories.

Different maps of the same terrain do not necessarily look alike, even when they are equally accurate. For one thing, the maps may be drawn to convey different information. There is no essential need to include political boundaries in a climatological or topographic map, no need to include highways in a map intended to guide high-altitude jets. Then they may be based on alternative organizing principles—recall how different things look in the various projections that are used to map the round earth onto a flat surface. These differences are not capricious, of course. Like the content, they are dictated by the use for which the maps are intended. Some projections are most suited for navigation; others work best for thematic maps illustrating population density or disease distribution.

Any map, geographic or psychic, must be evaluated according to how well it suits its intended purpose. Psychoanalytic models are judged by how well they map an underlying clinical sensibility. That is what I plan to do in this chapter. As my starting place I will take the tripartite structural model of the mind, first proposed by Freud and developed by his followers within the tradition of ego psychology, because it is the most evolved, articulated, and widely accepted map in the psychoanalytic literature. Most literate people, including analysts of widely disparate views, cannot discuss psychological issues for very long without speaking of

egos, superegos, and ids. The structural model guides and even gives shape to our deepest understanding of psychodynamic issues.

But the map is not the terrain, and despite its wide acceptance, I believe that Freud's model no longer adequately accounts for what we know clinically. I doubt, for that matter, that it ever accounted very well for what Freud himself knew clinically. The three agencies of the tripartite model embody a narrow facet of his vision of human nature—one that he felt passionately but that limits the scope of clinical inquiry. Because of this, we need to be aware of the sensibility contained within the model of which id, ego, and superego are components. Otherwise we are in danger of becoming unwittingly constrained by it.

Much of what I say has at least indirect relevance to the many alternative theories that have been proposed. There are no models of the mind that can stand up very well to the sort of analysis I will undertake. We do not have an adequate map in psychoanalysis today.

FROM his early division of the mind into the ego and the repressed through the later tripartite model, Freud proposed a number of psychic maps. Although they look quite different, they all represent attempts to model the workings of a mind divided by conflict. Freud's sensitivity to conflict is so embedded in psychoanalytic tradition that Ernst Kris could suggest that the very subject matter of psychoanalysis "is human behavior viewed as conflict" (1947, p. 6). Thus it can be difficult to keep in mind what a novel idea conflict is: it suggests that people are capable of constructing ideas that are so wildly incompatible that some of them must be banished from awareness.

Why should this be so? Why isn't it possible to think contradictory thoughts, to tolerate a range of impulses, or to accept the inevitability of emotional ambivalence? In his paper on "Repression," Freud raised these questions, which go to the core of any dynamic understanding of psychological life. Addressing the observation that wishes are often barred from consciousness, he asked:

> Why should an instinctual impulse undergo a vicissitude like this? A necessary condition of its happening must clearly be that the instinct's attainment of its aim should produce unpleasure instead of pleasure. But we cannot well imagine such a contingency. There are no such instincts: satisfaction of an instinct is always pleasurable. We should have to assume certain peculiar cir-

cumstances, some sort of process by which the pleasure of satisfaction is changed into unpleasure (1915b, p. 146).

The question is framed in the context of Freud's drive model, which presumes that repression is always directed against instinctually derived wishes. Its implications, however, can easily be extended to include the banishment from consciousness of any mental content—beliefs, perceptions, judgments, or self-observations.

What are the "peculiar circumstances" that make satisfaction of a wish (or awareness of any mental content) unpleasurable? Freud's several approaches to the problem are surprisingly vague. Nowhere in his work is there a vision of the motives underlying repression that is comparable in boldness or clinical utility to his theory of the instincts. This is alluded to but not clarified in the frequently heard assertion that, as his thinking evolved, he gave id psychology priority over ego psychology.

Any answer to Freud's question implies a particular vision of the conflicts that shape human experience. I believe that, over the course of his career, Freud addressed the problem in two quite different ways. First, he proposed that conflict arises when people are in danger of becoming aware of something about themselves that is incompatible with preferred—and therefore conscious—ideas. In contemporary psychoanalytic terms, conflict arises among highly discrepant self-representations. This view informed Freud's psychoanalytic theory and practice at its very beginning; there is evidence that he never entirely abandoned it. It faded, however, in the light of a second hypothesis: conflict is the inevitable consequence of the antagonism between human passions and the requirements of civilization. Originating (phylogenetically and ontogenetically) in generational strife, this conflict is internalized in the universal psychic struggle between the discharge of impulse and its prohibition.

Freud's two visions of the nature of conflict inevitably led him to two distinct theories of the motives that instigate repression. Although he was never explicit about these differences—Freud was rarely moved to articulate or contrast his various approaches to any issue—they underlie each of his models of the mind.

Repression and the Sense of Self

Freud's first approach to the problem of repression winds through the body of his writings; it can be abstracted from various texts as a sensibility.

In this version, repression is motivated by the need to maintain a continuing sense of the integrity and goodness of the self, an abiding belief in one's physical safety and in the stability of one's place in the interpersonal world. Repression is the guardian of the sense of self.

This sensibility appears in three different versions of the repressive process. Freud never integrated these versions into a single formulation. He could have done so because, although couched in different language and drawing on different observations, they are compatible. Their integration would have given rise to a powerful theory and would have avoided some of the difficulties of Freud's alternative view of conflict. I will briefly summarize each formulation.

1. Repression is instigated in order to isolate and preserve a particular set of ideas—those that dominate our conscious impressions of ourselves and our circumstances. This is the view of the early defense model (Freud, 1894, 1896b) and informed the clinical vision of *Studies on Hysteria* (Breuer and Freud, 1895). Freud acknowledged the dynamic role of "what is dominant in consciousness" as late as "Repression" (1915b, p. 152). He never found it necessary to articulate any complete list of the ideas that might be dominant in the mind of the individual, but they clearly involve maintaining a sense of self-integrity. Early on, Breuer and Freud prominently included threats to physical safety in their list of potentially pathogenic traumas (p. 9). Rapaport, reviewing the *Studies,* emphasized the psychological side of personal integrity, the need to maintain "social propriety and self-respect" (1959, p. 18).

2. Repression is organically motivated. Tied to the maturational emergence of psychosexual stages, the theory of organic repression suggests that what was experienced as a pleasure in one period is experienced with disgust or shame after the stage is transcended (Freud, 1950, letter 75; 1905a). Freud discusses organic repression as phylogenetically determined and operating strictly according to constitutional characteristics. Thus the concept itself is overbiologized and easily overlooked as void of psychological content—witness the term "organic repression" itself. But, as happens so often when he starts formulating things biologically, Freud quickly returns to psychology. The motive for repression is, accordingly, the *wish* to avoid the unpleasant feelings evoked by abandoned pleasures. The role of self-respect, carried over from the early defense model, is apparent in Freud's allusion to feelings of shame. Old pleasures must be repressed because they threaten feelings of self-regard that accompany developmen-

tal advance. Many years after proposing the theory of organic repression, years, in fact, after apparently having abandoned it, Freud echoed the early theory in purely psychological terms: "Man's archaic heritage forms the nucleus of the unconscious mind; and whatever part of that heritage has to be left behind in the advance to later phases of development, because it is unserviceable or incompatible with what is new and harmful to it, falls a victim to the process of repression" (1919, p. 204).

3. Repression operates in behalf of the ego instincts and of an ego motivated by narcissistic concerns. The aim of the ego instincts and (although less clearly developed) of narcissistic libido is organized around a desire to sustain the intactness of the self. Freud framed this mainly in terms of the body, using examples such as hunger, thirst, and the wish to maintain physical intactness by avoiding castration (1910c, 1916–17). Along with the theory of organic repression, this approach characterized Freud's thinking during the years when his drive model was at its height, before the structural theory returned him (partially) to the social sensibilities that informed his earliest views (see Greenberg and Mitchell, 1983, pp. 32–37). Society has virtually no impact on the workings of the ego instincts or on organic repression. In accord with the principles of the drive model, the motive for repression, like all motives and feelings, originates endogenously. But both of the later formulations trace the repressive process to needs to sustain personal well-being.

Clinically, the view that repression protects our sense of self is clearest in Freud's earliest vignettes. Examples in *Studies on Hysteria* include: a woman feeling angry about a companion who allows her dog to drink from a glass, yet wanting to be polite (Anna O.); a mother feeling afraid in a physically dangerous situation, yet wanting to keep up a calm appearance for the sake of her children (Frau Emmy von N.); and a young girl enjoying an exciting and romantic date, yet concerned about the health of her father (Fraulein Elisabeth von R.). Correspondingly, a wide range of emotions arises from the failure to preserve a sense of physical and psychological well-being. Among others, Breuer and Freud (1895) emphasize fright, anxiety, shame, physical pain, pain over a lost relationship, and social humiliation.

This interpretive perspective continues, with few changes, in *The Interpretation of Dreams*. In the dream analyses he presents there, Freud talks about conflicting wishes, a narrower category theoretically than the incompatible ideas of the *Studies*. But when we ask the next, clinically crucial

question—what, exactly, is wished for?—we are back on familiar ground. Both the ideas of the 1895 and the wishes of 1900 turn on preserving a valued sense of self.

Consider Freud's interpretation of the "specimen dream of psychoanalysis," Irma's injection:

> The conclusion of the dream . . . was that I was not responsible for the persistence of Irma's pains . . . The dream acquitted me of the responsibility for Irma's condition . . . The dream represented a particular state of affairs as I should have wished it to be. *Thus its content was the fulfilment of a wish and its motive was a wish* (1900, pp. 118–119).

Again, analyzing the famous dream of the botanical monograph:

> the dream . . . turns out to have been in the nature of a self-justification, a plea on behalf of my own rights . . . What it meant was: "After all, I'm the man who wrote the valuable and memorable paper (on cocaine)" . . . what I was insisting was: "I may allow myself to do this" (p. 173).

The wishes responsible for these dreams, two of the most thoroughly analyzed in the book, aim at maintaining a self-image that has been threatened by Freud's concerns about his actions.

Psychic Conflict and Structural Models

When psychoanalytic theorists map the mind, they divide the terrain into units called psychic structures. The use of a term like structure, with its connotation of physical presence, does not simply reflect a wished-for bridge to anatomy, physics, or the other hard sciences. More important, it embodies our belief in the stability of human psychology. Because we can talk about structure, we can talk about pattern and sequence. This allows us to navigate clinically using at least an approximate guide, to generalize about what we have seen, and to communicate our findings to others. If psychoanalysis is to be a theory and not just a set of observations, it must have some construct that captures the continuity within the flux of human life.

All psychoanalytic definitions of structure begin with the idea of stability: psychic structures resist change and endure over time. Rapaport, certainly the great anatomist of psychoanalysis, said that we use the term to mean "a relatively stable . . . characteristic configuration that we can abstract from the behavior observed" (1967, p. 701). And even Sullivan,

archenemy of the reifications abounding in post-Freudian ego psychology, recognized a need to cover conceptually similar terrain. Importing the term "dynamism" from philosophy (and from medicine as well), he defined it as "the relatively enduring pattern of energy transformations which recurrently characterize the organism in its duration as a living organism" (1953, p. 103).

But should *all* enduring mental organizations be defined as structures? Consider characteristic fantasies, behavioral reaction patterns, motives, capacities of various kinds, and self and object representations. Each is relatively stable and resilient in the face of changing circumstances. But they are not structures in the fullest sense because they do not explain the occurrence of psychological events. A further distinction is needed: within any theoretical system we must differentiate organizations that carry out a psychological function from those that do not. Only functional organizations qualify as psychic structures; the rest are simply stable and persistent mental contents (Hartmann, Kris, and Loewenstein, 1946; F. Schwartz, 1981; Pulver, 1988).

The distinction between psychic contents and psychic functions is crucial and must be maintained. Yet it can give the impression that psychoanalysis needs to straddle the psychological world of experience and the biological world of mechanism. My analogy with maps casts a different light on the problem. I have said that maps of the mind, like their geographic counterparts, are shaped both by their creator's observations and by the organizing principles that have been applied. These organizing principles reflect a particular solution to the problem of extracting order from (some would say imposing order upon) the endlessly intricate flow of human experience. Only after arriving at a conceptual framework for doing so—frameworks typically invoking concepts such as drives, relationships, or self-development—does it make sense to draw the kinds of boundaries that define psychic units.

So theorists must develop an interpretive stance before they can formulate structural models. That is where function enters the picture. Precisely *because* they are presumed to function, these structures *explain* the qualities of experience that the theorist is trying to capture. Functioning units of the mind fulfill an essential theoretical role: they embody—literally—an analyst's fundamental clinical sensibility.

This is why there are so many different structural models. Kohut's bipolar self reflects the assumption that development aims toward the achievement of stable goals and ideals and that, if achieved, these can serve

as a compass for steering a satisfying course through life's difficulties. Fairbairn, in contrast, derived his structural theory from a "basic endopsychic situation" based on the vicissitudes of the child's early object seeking. His model of an ego split into three parts, each tied inextricably to an object representation, embodies the developing child's attempts to connect with a sometimes loved, sometimes hated, but always needed caretaker. Sullivan, notwithstanding his aversion to structural concepts, has a diagram labeled "Schematic of Personality" that is organized around degrees of anxiety. This in turn ramifies into a very structurelike depiction of interpersonal relationships based on areas of anxiety in the personalities of the participants (1964, pp. 239–246).

As FREUD's clinical views evolved, he proposed several structural models. Each must be evaluated on the basis of how well it maps the sorts of conflicts that shape human experience generally and psychopathology in particular. Arlow and Brenner have expressed the same thought in different words:

> If we are to divide the mental apparatus into separate parts, the division must be along the lines of cleavage which are apparent in conflict; otherwise our theoretical division is of no use to us just where we need it the most in our practice. What we need in our practice is a theory that will help us to understand, to study, and to treat situations of intrapsychic conflict (1964, p. 28).

Two of Freud's models have been given formal names that reflect their quasi-geographic character—the topographic model of 1900 and the tripartite structural model of 1923. Some of the others were never formally named, but guided psychoanalytic thinking for considerable periods of time. A mind divided into the conscious ego and the repressed, which evolved during the early 1890's, was the first. Still others, less completely developed, were designed as stopgaps to solve specific clinical problems. The clearest example of this is the topographic model as it stood between 1914 and 1923, supplemented by the ego and the ego ideal. These structures fit uncomfortably into the topographic model itself, which was supposed to map the entire terrain of the mind. But they were needed to account for Freud's (and Abraham's) otherwise inexplicable ideas about narcissism (Freud, 1914a) and depression (Freud, 1917a).

Freud's earliest model of the mind most clearly embodies his view that conflict arises when belief in the well-being or goodness of the self is threatened. In *Studies on Hysteria,* the conscious ego is a collection of

ideas; he defined it as the "dominant mass of ideas." Any idea (thought, perception, belief, memory, impulse, fantasy) that was compatible with the dominant mass of ideas could become and remain conscious. Any idea that was significantly incompatible with the ego became a candidate for repression. It is interesting that in the *Studies* Freud talks about the repression of ideas, although his examples involve impulses (sexual or vengeful, typically) and affects (fear, disgust, and so on). Apparently he was concerned with impulses and affects mainly as they became manifest in ideas about the self. Preferred ideas about the self could be contaminated by an unacceptable thought (a socially inappropriate sexual or vengeful impulse) or by an unwelcome feeling (fear or disgust). Freud's 1895 model, accordingly, divided the mind into a region containing personally acceptable self representations (the ego, or the dominant mass of ideas) and a region containing warded-off, potentially toxic ideas (the repressed).

When commentators trace the evolution of Freud's various structural models, the formulation of 1895 is often overlooked. Certainly this was a roughly drawn model. I have already mentioned that he merely alluded to what the dominant ideas were. Further, the model contains no hint about the structure's developmental history. Freud never discussed the ontogeny of the conscious ego; he was silent about how the dominant mass of ideas got to be dominant. Moreover, the ego's role in the psychic economy was more narrowly sketched than it was to be in the structural model of 1923. There was nothing like the extended list of ego functions that we have come to associate with that structure as we think of it today. Its one function was to act as the guardian of conscious awareness.

But it is misleading to dismiss Freud's intent in the *Studies* to formulate a working model of the mind. Despite its narrowness and lack of a history, the ego of 1895 is clearly a mental structure. It meets the defining criteria of stability and function. In fact, the one function attributed to it—defense—was the key factor in explaining the pathogenesis of the psychoneuroses. The model of 1895 satisfies the requirements of the Arlow and Brenner quote cited above: it explains conflict as conflict was understood at the time.

The topographic model, introduced in *The Interpretation of Dreams* and amplified in the metapsychological papers of 1915–1917, is generally considered Freud's first developed map of the mind. Certainly the topographic model is more complex and elaborate than the sketchy map of the *Studies*. It spells out crucial distinctions between the operation of conscious and unconscious mental processes, it addresses the functions of

three "regions" of the mind, and it attempts to explain the dynamic interaction of conscious and unconscious contents.

These differences in sophistication, however, tend to obscure what I think may be a more important continuity between the two maps. The topographic model is a far more intricate system because it is more explicit about how repression works. That is, it elaborates the functional side of model making. Much simpler is its approach to the question of why repression should be necessary. When Freud speaks to this point, his views are little changed from what they had been earlier. In *The Interpretation of Dreams* repression is carried out by the censor, a substructure within the preconscious system. Freud says little about what motivates the censor, except to suggest that it operates as the "watchman of our mental health" (1900, p. 567). With further development of the topographic model, the censor apparently works on behalf of the ego ideal, which itself is the center of what Freud calls "self-regard" (1914a, p. 100). The purpose of repression is to avoid ideas that would be incompatible with ongoing feelings of self-regard. From this point of view, things are much as they were in the earliest formulation.

The most explicit statement about the motives of the censor that I have been able to find occurs in lecture 9 of Freud's *Introductory Lectures:* "The purposes which exercise the censorship are those which are acknowledged by the dreamer's waking judgement, *those with which he feels himself at one* . . . The purposes against which the dream-censorship is directed must be described . . . from the point of view of [the censor] itself . . . they are invariably of a reprehensible nature, repulsive from the ethical, aesthetic and social point of view—matters of which one does not venture to think at all or thinks only with disgust" (1916–17, p. 142, my italics).

The idea of judgments "with which he feels himself at one" is remarkably like a conscious ego made up of a dominant mass of ideas. This sense of self is threatened by what Freud in the next sentence strikingly (and somewhat confusingly) calls "an unbridled and ruthless egoism." He gives a few examples of such threatening thoughts; they include lust, hatred, and wishes for revenge (p. 143). The possible confusion—between judgments based on self-regard and egoism—is clarified if we reflect on the tone of Freud's remarks. The description sounds judgmental. It is as if one person is looking down, contemptuously, on another. This suggests to me that, as in the earlier model, Freud is describing a conflict among ideas about the self. The censor, like the earlier ego, somewhat harshly reviews various motives as they are embodied in self-representations. Some are

deemed acceptable and become components of conscious self-regard; many are condemned as reprehensible or disgusting and suffer repression. The topographic theory, like the model of 1895, explains conflicts among peoples' alternative visions of themselves.

Repression in the Drive Model

Freud worked with the topographic model for twenty-three years, longer than he held on to any other map of the mind. It supports the broad view of conflict that opened the way to psychoanalytic treatment and informed the clinical material of *Studies on Hysteria*. But the seeds of its destruction were planted when Freud arrived at his drive model in 1905. In the early drive theory a momentous assumption was made: the *only* mental contents that are inadmissible to consciousness are libidinally driven wishes. Correspondingly, the only motive for repression is an inherent antagonism between drive and ego, or between the discharge of impulse and its prohibition.

This view of conflict is very different from the one I have been discussing. First, within the terms of the drive model, the only sort of mental content that can instigate conflict is a wishful impulse. Second, the only source of a wishful impulse is sexuality. In the earlier theory, memories, perceptions, beliefs, and such could also generate conflict. Now they cannot unless they are bound to sexual impulses. Repression, Freud wrote at the end of his life, can be directed only against "the component instincts of sexual life" (1940, p. 186).* The implication of the dual-instinct theory of course, and this is borne out by Freud's clinical use of it, is that aggressive impulses are also candidates for repression (and for the other vicissitudes of instinct). Still Freud persisted in references to libido alone as subject to repression; not until Hartmann did a Freudian analyst redress this peculiar omission (Greenberg, 1986).

The topographic model does not adequately map the more restricted view of conflict embodied in the drive theory. Recall that the model was designed to explain the way a mental content—*any* mental content—moved between conscious and unconsciousness. But when Freud nar-

---

*In fairness I should point out that when Freud still held to the seduction theory—long before the advent of his drive model—he wrote that "only ideas with a sexual content can be repressed" (1896b, p. 167n). But then his view of repression was much more narrowly tied to its role in the etiology of the transference neuroses; I believe it deserves less weight than the later formulations.

rowed his conception of the forces involved in conflict, then one of the structures in any model of conflict must have an essential and unalterable connection with sexuality. The unconscious (systemic Ucs.) has no such connection. Although it is associated with the infantile and with wishful thinking, nothing in its formulation even suggests that its contents are exclusively sexual.

Further, the hypothesis that only a libidinal impulse can be repressed implies an intriguing corollary: repression must be instigated by something that opposes *only* sexual ideas. Consider how this would affect Freud's early structural theories. The dominant mass of ideas, those constituting the ego, no longer is organized around feelings of physical and psychological well-being. Instead it is exclusively antisexual. And what of the preconscious censor? As custodian of the sense of self, it casts too wide a net to be the specific opponent of sexuality. Can the guardian of mental health see threats to sanity arising solely from sensual urges? Where once repression served the need to maintain a sense of personal integrity and goodness, now it is based on a puritanical abhorrence of passion.

What is there in human nature that stands in fundamental opposition to the demands of sexuality *but to nothing else?* At times Freud himself seemed daunted by the difficulty of conceptualizing this in motivational terms. He was led to describe a conflict "between suppressed erotism and the forces that were keeping it in repression" (1907, p. 52). Or, in a later and more general formulation, to suggest that dreams and neurotic symptoms "are compromises between the demands of a repressed impulse and the resistance of a censoring force in the ego" (1925b, p. 45). In both statements there is a motive on one side of the conflict, opposed by a motiveless force on the other.

The idea that a repressive *force* opposes a threatening *motive* is not a satisfactory solution to Freud's problem. It is conceptually inconsistent because it depicts a conflict between an idea (the motive) on the one hand and a quasi-physical quantity (the force) on the other. There can be no such conflict because ideas and forces are concepts drawn from different universes of discourse. As such, they cannot conflict with (or for that matter be in harmony with) each other; they cannot meet in any way.*

Freud and many of his followers within the ego-psychological tradition

---

*The various formulations are fine examples of what the philosopher Gilbert Ryle (1949) called a "category mistake"—the forced joining of ideas drawn from different conceptual categories. One might as well say, "The football collided with Thursday."

attempted to resolve this inconsistency by giving motive a physical basis: libido itself is a quantity that has momentum and exerts force. So the parties to conflict on both sides are physical entities. But the solution doesn't work, at least from the perspective of the questions I am raising.* It fails because, once Freud turned away from his view that repression was the guardian of self-respect, he offered no adequate *psychological* account of the threat posed by the drives. Thus his dramatic illumination of the life of the impulses has no counterpart in his motivational analysis of the defenses. And yet every analyst knows, as Peter Gay has said succinctly, that a defense is also a wish (1985, p. 110). Analytic understanding requires that we know the motive for any wish, whether its aim is instinctual gratification or defense. Despite this, a great deal of psychoanalytic theorizing has been haunted by the supposed clash between ideas and forces.

Freud's search for the motive that opposes our awareness of instinctual impulses led to one of his most characteristic and most revolutionary theoretical premises. The antagonist of sexuality and destructiveness, he came to believe, is not an endogenous motive such as maintaining an intact sense of self. There is nothing inherent in human nature that requires the repression of *anything*.† Rather, the opposition is imposed from outside; it is a requirement of society. Phylogenetically, social relations among people became possible only after the forced renunciation of incestuous and parricidal strivings (Freud, 1912–13, 1987). This is repeated ontogenetically, by everybody. Each person's crowning developmental achievement—the passage from self-centered, impulse-ridden infancy to individuated living in the broader human community—depends on this renunciation. The nuclear conflict in human life is between the unmodulated expression of innate impulse and the social unacceptability of such expression.

The structural theory outlined in *The Ego and the Id* did not yet quite support this vision of conflict. The model was fully developed only with Freud's revised theory of the relation between repression and anxiety.

---

*A similar observation has been made, on rather different grounds, by some of the most trenchant critics of Freud's metapsychology—most notably Merton Gill, George Klein, and Roy Schafer. Also relevant is a series of brilliant papers by Bernard Apfelbaum (1962, 1965, 1966), who has criticized the weakening of motivational theorizing in the structural model, especially in its elaboration in the work of Hartmann, Rapaport, and other ego psychologists.

†Anna Freud (1936) wrote about an inherent antagonism between the ego and the drives. In a similar vein, Rapaport (1951) discussed premotivational conflict based on structural differences in rates of discharge. But these emendations of Freud's vision lack the sorts of clinical implications that psychoanalytic theories require.

Now Freud argued that anxiety is not, as he earlier believed, the consequence of failed repression. Instead, repression is necessary when an impulse arouses the anticipation of danger, as signaled by feelings of anxiety. And the source of danger can always be traced back to the outside world. "The ego," Freud wrote, "is threatened by dangers which come *in the first instance* from external reality" (1940, p. 199, my italics). The sequence of five danger situations that Freud spelled out in *Inhibitions, Symptoms and Anxiety* (1926) alludes to threats to the self. The nature of the threats changes as the child develops, but the first four of them—birth, loss of the mother, loss of the mother's love, and castration—are disasters of external origin. The final, developmentally open-ended danger—the potential loss of the superego's love—is at first glance entirely endopsychic. But ultimately the source of the danger is environmental, since once formed the superego plays "the part of an external world for the ego" (Freud, 1940, p. 206).

It is a central tenet of Freud's revised anxiety theory that environmental dangers do not arise randomly and are not predominantly a function of the character of other people in the child's interpersonal world. Although "the instinctual situation which is feared goes back ultimately to an external situation of danger" (1933, p. 89), we would not be threatened "if we did not entertain certain feelings and intentions within us" (1926, p. 145). In light of this, the capacity for repression evolved as an adaptive response to societal hostility to the instincts. This process is repeated in the experience of every growing child, particularly in parental retaliation for oedipal wishes.

MANY analysts mistakenly believe that the tripartite model accounts for conflict in some generic way. Arlow, for one, suggests that the model "was devised precisely for the purpose of organizing and clarifying the phenomenology of mental life as consequences of conflict" (1985b, p. 22). And Boesky argues that the very concept of structure itself is "codefined by intrapsychic conflict" (1988, p. 118). But these authors fail to realize that the structural theory does not *simply* account for conflict. Virtually any model of a divided mind can do that, and by 1923 Freud had published and rejected at least two other mental topographies. But the vision of neurotic conflict embodied in the tripartite model as elaborated by the revised theory of anxiety is very specific: conflict derives from the antagonism between a person's innate endowment and external social circumstances.

1. On a broad, philosophical level, the conflict is between human nature,

the product of our phylogenetic heritage, and society. "It is quite impossible," Freud wrote, "to adjust the claims of the sexual instinct to the demands of civilization" (1912b, p. 190). Having thus framed the problem, he proceeds in the pessimistic tradition of Hobbes, suggesting in *The Future of an Illusion* that "every individual is virtually an enemy of civilization" (1927, p. 6) and in *Civilization and Its Discontents* that civilization "is built up upon a renunciation of instinct" (1930, p. 97).

2. From a biological perspective, developed from Freud's writings by Hartmann and his followers in ego psychology, the conflict is between instinct and adaptation. Man's instincts, Hartmann wrote, are alienated from reality in a way that the instincts of animals are not (1939a, p. 48), and the ego emerges as a "very highly differentiated organ of adaptation" (1939b, p. 13).

3. Clinically, the conflict is between the spontaneous expression of impulse and inhibition of that expression in order to avoid danger originally experienced as coming from the outside world. "Just as the id is directed exclusively to obtaining pleasure," Freud writes, "so the ego is governed by considerations of safety" (1940, p. 199). And safety is difficult to attain, largely because the ego "has to defend its existence against an external world which threatens it with annihilation" (p. 200). In the course of development, this entire conflict becomes internalized so that, as Hartmann and Loewenstein put it, "regulations that have taken place in interaction with the outside world are replaced by inner regulations" (1962, p. 150).

Structural Models, Procrustean Beds

Freud's revised vision of human conflict is brooding, brilliant, and compelling to anyone who has struggled with an experienced gulf between private and social living. It is also, clinically, a strikingly narrow perspective, because it is weak at conceptualizing the *content* of the conflicts that matter most.

First it is assumed that the parties to conflict are always impulses and something that opposes their satisfaction. Then there is a presumption that impulses originate internally, in bodily (or endopsychic) stirrings that may be serendipitously stimulated by external events but that in any case would follow their own intrinsic rhythm. The prohibition, in sharp contrast, always originates in environmental constraints deriving from the societal condemnation of human passions.

Consider the idea that impulse and prohibition always represent the

poles of a conflict. This assumption fails to capture the way conflict plays out in clinical work. In the course of any good analysis, a wide range of conflicts will occupy center stage at different times. Some of these will involve subjectively incompatible personal goals: a desire for autonomy and fear of losing the comfort that comes with feelings of closeness; the need to trust one's reality testing while being afraid of the security that comes with having the world explained and interpreted by somebody else; the desire to pursue ambitious goals while holding on to cherished feelings of youth and helplessness. Often we will see conflicts centered on specific interpersonal attachments: irreconcilable loyalties to the two parents; or ambivalent feelings directed toward the same person (for example, wishes to separate from a person one also needs).

The list of conflicts with which analysts regularly work is inexhaustible. Many of those mentioned are of the sort that Anton Kris (1984) has called "conflicts of ambivalence," in contrast to the more familiar "conflicts of defense." None of them falls comfortably into the impulse/prohibition polarity. One potential solution to the problem would be simply to ignore the model when the clinical material exceeds its scope. We would occasionally be without a map but so, after all, are all explorers. I believe that some (perhaps many) analysts actually work this way. But there is a more insidious problem. The structural theory, like all models, influences the very way we perceive the phenomena it purports to explain.

In a passage criticizing the applicability of the tripartite structural model to the psychology of early childhood, John Gedo writes, "until the acquisition of a structured morality, the child's hierarchy of aims does not create intrapsychic conflict" (1979, p. 226). This is an extraordinary triumph of presumption over observation. Almost as soon as we can see motives in children, we can see incompatibility and conflict among them. The ambivalent child at the anal stage (or the rapprochement subphase, or just the terrible twos) is paradigmatic, though this is certainly not the earliest example. But it is not true conflict *as defined in the terms of the structural model*. For Gedo, and for many other analysts, the model has become a procrustean bed rather than a heuristic tool. It prescribes what we define as conflict—and therefore what we seek out in doing the work of analysis—rather than modeling conflict as we see it clinically.

Analysts working closely within the confines of the structural model must assume that one side of a conflict is *always* a defense. Fenichel put it this way: "The neurotic conflict, by definition, is one between a tendency striving for discharge and another tendency that tries to prevent this dis-

charge" (1945, p. 129). More recently, Brenner has expressed a similar view: "Drive derivatives conflict only when one is used to ward off another ... What is important to realize is that they are in conflict because one is used defensively to ward the other off in order to eliminate or to alleviate unpleasure" (1982, p. 34).

With this formulation Brenner arrives at a remarkable conclusion. He suggests that conflict "was not truly central to Freud's theory of neurosogenesis prior to 1926" (1982, p. 6). Surely it is clear, from all that has been said so far, that Freud's conflict theory was not only central but most powerful before his introduction of the drive model in 1905. Brenner's view is plausible only if we agree that nothing but impulses and prohibitions can come into conflict with each other. Once we agree, we have constructed a circular argument. Far more important, we have put on clinical blinders.

Anticipating the objection that limiting conflict to an antagonism between impulse and defense (ego and id) artificially constrains the psychoanalytic vision, Fenichel went on to discuss whether there can be conflicts between different instinctual demands. He based his answer on one of the central elements in Freud's definition of the id, that it knows nothing of contradiction. Because of this, Fenichel argues, "if the history of conflicts of this type is investigated it is regularly *found* that the apparent conflict between instincts merely covers or represents another conflict between an undesirable instinct and some fear or guilt feeling that objects" (1945, pp. 129–130, my italics; see also Brenner, 1982, pp. 33–34). Notice that Fenichel passes this off as an empirical finding. I doubt that it would accord with the experience of many analysts but, beyond that, it is not really a finding at all: it is an assumption about what will be found that determines clinical sensibilities and interpretive content.

Gedo, Brenner, and Fenichel have a sound if somewhat fundamentalist (Schafer, 1988) understanding of the vision of conflict embodied in the tripartite model. Their view is supported by what Freud said about the ontogeny of the three agencies. While any formulation is necessarily a simplification, it can be put this way: within the terms of the structural model as originally conceived, the id is connected to the body and represents its hypothesized instinctual needs; the superego is connected to an essentially hostile external world and represents its prohibitions; the ego is connected to perceptual processes and represents a need to balance internal and external demands. As a result, the id can *only* want, the superego can *only* judge, and the ego can *only* mediate and create compromise solu-

tions. The content of human conflict inevitably must involve a struggle between impulse and the need to control it.

THE TRIPARTITE model further limits our vision of conflict by tracing the origin of impulses exclusively to endogenous sources while assigning prohibitions exclusively to environmental constraint. I have already referred to Freud's Hobbesian pessimism about the inherent incompatibility between human nature and society. Like other aspects of his conflict theory, this grew out of the drive model. Consider the differences between the ego of *Studies on Hysteria* and the ego of drive theory. The ego of 1895, the dominant mass of ideas, is exquisitely social. The sense of well-being that the ego works so hard to preserve is intimately bound up with maintaining a benign connection with the interpersonal world. It is essentially tied to the human environment. Freud did not dwell on this tie in interpersonal or developmental terms. He apparently thought it self-evident that the individual would draw sustenance and a personal sense of satisfaction from fitting in with social reality (Apfelbaum, 1965, 1966).

In stark contrast, the ego of the tripartite model is fundamentally narcissistic. Its role in the psychic economy is to facilitate as much instinctual gratification as possible while avoiding the dangers of doing so. Freud put it this way in *New Introductory Lectures:* "the ego . . . has taken on the task of representing the external world to the id—fortunately for the id, which could not escape destruction if, in its blind efforts for the satisfaction of its instincts, it disregarded that supreme external power" (1933, p. 75). This narcissism underlies the ego's delicate psychic balancing act. Freud sometimes sounds as if he were describing the posturing of a misbehaving child nervously trying to cover his own tracks: the ego "*clothes* the id's . . . commands with . . . rationalizations; it *pretends* that the id is showing obedience to the admonitions of reality . . . it *disguises* the id's conflicts with reality" (1923a, p. 56, my italics).

When social influence enters the intrapsychic equation, it is not carried by the ego of the tripartite model, but by the superego. And, because Freud assumed that society is fundamentally hostile toward the drives, the narcissistic ego is in an adversarial relationship with its intrapsychic neighbor:

> The torments caused by the reproaches of conscience correspond precisely to a child's fear of loss of love, a fear the place of which has been taken by the moral agency . . . In this way the super-ego continues to play the part of an

external world for the ego, although it has become a portion of the internal world. Throughout later life it represents the influence of a person's childhood, of the care and education given him by his parents (1940, p. 206).

Notice the way Freud has shifted his emphasis. Previously he had spoken of an ego that looks to society as guarantor of an innate need to preserve a sense of self. Now he refers to fears of society in general and of the parents in particular. Left to our own devices, anything goes. It is only the requirements of others that persuade us to turn our back on even the most outlandish impulses. If we do not kill, rape, or rob, it is only because we are afraid. The ego rejects the id's impulses because, narcissistically, it fears the people who oppose them.

When analysts do recognize the narrowness of the vision of conflict in the tripartite model, what we typically get is a dazzling display of metapsychological acrobatics, all designed to save the basic framework. Consider: intrasystemic conflict, a structured id, adapted aspects of the drives, superego precursors, the blurring of impulse-defense distinctions, neutralization, the conflict-free sphere, primary ego energy, primary undifferentiated energy, primary autonomy, secondary autonomy, and more. Applying each of these concepts to the interpretive system of psychoanalysis broadens our vision of the forces implicated in conflict, or defines areas of psychological functioning that are exempt from the impulse/prohibition antithesis. At the same time, each also contributes to making psychoanalytic theory unwieldy and internally contradictory.

An example from David Rapaport's writings illustrates how one ego-psychological emendation of the structural view of conflict—the idea of secondary autonomy (Hartmann, 1939a, 1950)—would affect clinical interpretation. Rapaport's discussion highlights both the problem that had to be addressed and the strained clinical perspective that emerges from its solution.

Rapaport discusses altruism as an example of how a motive may become secondarily autonomous. In Freud's 1895 model, although he doesn't mention it explicitly, altruistic feelings and actions can be assumed to be part of man's inherently social nature. The dominant mass of ideas must include altruism. With the advent of the new model of drive and structures, however, altruism cannot be a primary motive because it is neither pleasure-seeking nor destructive. Instead it must arise as a defensive transformation of some asocial (even antisocial) tendency. Rapaport recognized the interpretive constraints of this idea but could not abandon the assumption of the model. Thus he invoked secondary autonomy:

many altruistic . . . motivations are somehow related to reaction formations against impulses of the anal-sadistic phase . . . [But] altruism as a motivating *value*—though it arose as a reaction formation or an altruistic denial—need not be lost, and is mostly not lost, in successful analyses.

To generalize this point: what came about as a result of conflict sooner or later may become independent of the conflict, may become relatively autonomous (1951, p. 364).

Here Rapaport perpetuates the fundamental assumption of the tripartite model: only instinctual impulses can become embroiled in conflict. Unless altruistic feelings are aimed specifically at the expression of sadistic impulses, they must be autonomous, outside conflict. How would this apply in a commonplace clinical situation, in patients' experience of conflict between their concern for others and their personal ambition? Following the dictates of the structural model, Rapaport saw two possibilities. Either the conflict revolves around a reaction-formation against the sadism that drives the patient's ambition, or there is no conflict at all.

This misses a central clinical point. Altruism may conflict with (and defend against) sadism, but it also may conflict with ambition on many other grounds. Altruism can be based on identification with a self-sacrificing mother, thus warding off the fears over separation that would come with fully realized ambitions. Or it can originate in loyalty to a particularly vulnerable father, one whom the patient learns would truly be injured by his son's success. These are simply two of a virtually limitless range of possibilities. They are the sorts of conflicts that every analyst knows about and should work with. There is, however, no way of conceptualizing them within the terms of the tripartite structural model, except as derivatives of putatively more fundamental conflicts.

Many analysts who are aware of the difficulties inherent in the structural model have tried to modify it by relying heavily on the concept of intrasystemic conflict. Also introduced by Hartmann (1950, 1951), it was designed to account for observed conflicts that could not be explained by the opposing activity of the three psychic agencies. Hartmann cites the typical ambivalence that patients have about following the fundamental rule. He conceptualizes this as a conflict between two ego functions: free associating and exercising control. Subsequently, a number of authors have invoked the concept of intrasystemic conflict to explain a great many of the phenomena that are at the center of clinical psychoanalytic interest (Rothstein, 1983; A. Kris, 1977, 1984).

The possibility of intrasystemic conflict solves the problems I have been

describing. It eliminates the assumption of the tripartite model that there is always an impulse on one side of the conflict and a prohibition on the other, and it no longer mandates the internal/external split. It allows for conflict between various mental contents (ideas, for instance, or self representations) or, as in Hartmann' early example, between wishes to exercise different ego functions. Rapaport's discussion of altruism and ambition (written before intrasystemic conflict was widely applied clinically) fits well into the idea that there are incompatible values held within the ego or the ego ideal. Unfortunately, the concept of intrasystemic conflict also destroys the theory it is designed to preserve. Recall what Arlow and Brenner said about drawing maps of the mind: "the division must be along the lines of cleavage which are apparent in conflict" (1964, p. 28). If there are conflicts that cannot be explained by these lines of cleavage, then why divide the mind into these particular three agencies in the first place? As far as I can tell, the theoretical emendation has rendered them vestigial. Inserting intrasystemic conflict into Freud's structural model is a classic example of a successful operation that killed the patient.

THE TRIPARTITE structural model has been a powerful force in the past six decades of psychoanalysis. But we have learned a great deal, and it no longer serves us well. Its Hobbesian vision of the unbridgeable gulf between innate motives and the requirements imposed upon us by society skews our appreciation of human conflict. We must leave it behind and challenge ourselves to model conflict in a way that reflects contemporary clinical experience. The new map would take two fundamental premises as its starting point:

1. Psychoanalysis, both as a theory and as a clinical method, begins with the observation that human experience is warped by peoples' perceived need to remain unaware of certain mental contents. This need is based on a belief that these contents would threaten the integrity of one's sense of self and consequently the feeling of safety and well-being. Therefore, consonant with Freud's earliest models, the primary distinction that must be retained is between those contents that are accessible to consciousness and those that are not. This distinction bears directly on our understanding of psychoanalytic treatment, which works by facilitating the patient's ability to expand the realm of consciousness by risking awareness of previously disavowed contents.

2. All mental contents, whether accessible to consciousness or not, are complex constructions containing both endogenous and perceptual ele-

ments. The structural model can make it difficult to keep in mind what most of us know: all impulses have social determinants, and all prohibitions are partly innate. In contrast, I suggest again that Freud was on the right track early on, when he talked about ideas. Ideas are constructed out of wishes, fears, experiences of the self and of others that are the residue of interpersonal exchanges, and a wide range of affective states that are part and parcel of all of these. It is useful to conceptualize mental contents as ideas or, in more contemporary terms, as representations (Sandler and Rosenblatt, 1962; Sandler and Sandler, 1987). In Sandler's definition, representations are not passive renderings of the person's situation, but are the multiply determined creations of an active mind.

What we need, then, is a model that embodies our understanding of the formation of mental representations and of the dynamic relationships—especially the incompatibility and ultimately the conflicts—among them. The model must include a vision of people actively constructing the elements of their representational world and selecting what will guide their experience. Because the goal of psychoanalytic treatment is to facilitate the patient's ability to risk increasing awareness of previously warded-off representations, the model must have implications for understanding the conditions needed for this increased awareness.

Wish, Affect, Representation

IN THIS chapter and the next I am going to work toward developing a psychoanalytic model that reflects clinical process as I understand it. My aim is not to construct a full-blown model of the mind; despite Freud's theoretical optimism, I doubt that the clinical psychoanalyst has the data to support any such undertaking. What I will do is to offer a model of the mental contents and the dynamic relationships among them that come into play in the course of struggling, along with our patients, to make the unconscious conscious.

Whenever authors set out to construct a psychoanalytic model, they begin by proposing a structure that embodies something essential in their clinical sensibility. Generally this central structure is presumed to exist prior to experience; a person is born with it, or at least with some prototype of it. The primordial structure for Freud was the id, the container of the passions that he thought gave direction to all mental activity. For Fairbairn it was the pristine ego, unconflicted in its need for objects. For Kohut it was the rudimentary self, striving toward the actualization and expression of personal potential. The possibilities go on. Even an apparently technical abstraction like Hartmann's undifferentiated matrix expresses a clinical vision: we are not all id at the beginning, because we are not simply creatures of blind passion; we are also creatures of adaptation.

My model is based on the assumptions I have relied on throughout this book: it maps the mind of people who are the agents of their behavior and experience, who struggle with conflicting goals and feelings, and whose fantasies play an important role in everything that happens psychologically. I will describe a mind that is inherently and unalterably active. It has considerable imaginative capabilities, which give meaning to all lived

experience in accord with the dictates of fundamental human needs. It is a mind whose contents can be intolerably conflicted, so much so that some elements must be tenaciously kept out of awareness.

Because my clinical commitment is focused on activity and personal agency, I begin with a structure that is capable of receiving stimuli, constructing and storing the representations that are the stuff of personal experience, formulating and choosing among alternative courses of action, and initiating action according to an evolved plan. Each of these may take place either consciously or unconsciously; awareness is a function of the structure, and repression is one of its capacities.

In beginning like this I am working within a well-established psychoanalytic tradition; many others have begun their theorizing by searching for the active core in the life of the mind. Thus there are similarities between the structure I am proposing and the self in Kohut's strongest definition of the term: the self, he wrote, is "a center of initiative and a recipient of impressions" (1977, p. 99). This broadly sketches the functions I have in mind, although his concept of the self includes many implications that I cannot accept—mainly his understanding of the fundamental goals of the self (see Chapter 4) and the patterns he finds most salient in both normal and pathological development. George Klein, like Kohut, saw the self as "a center to which activity is referred" (1976, p. 266). I owe much to Klein's thinking, although I believe that his personal contribution would have been clearer had he been less concerned with his own identity as a Freudian.

There is some overlap between what I am describing and Schafer's (1976) "I" or "person," defined as the agent of behavior and experience. Also, there are resemblances between my formulation and the synthetic function of the ego (Nunberg, 1930) and the adaptive ego (Hartmann, 1939a) of the classical structural model, as well as points of convergence with Sullivan's self system (1953). Perhaps the structure I have in mind is most like the ego that Freud described prior to his introduction of the drive model. Like that early ego, I am proposing a structure that is a container of ideas and that navigates a course through life based on the nature of those ideas.

The similarities to other models raise an irksome terminological question: what should the new structure be called? The "self" quickly comes to mind, but there are two compelling arguments against it. First, it has become politicized and something of a proprietary commodity "con-

trolled" by Kohut's followers. I would have to spend as much time saying what I don't mean about the structure as about what I do mean.

Second, and more important, in all its psychoanalytic incarnations the term has been used because it is close to experience; we all talk about and feel that we have a self of one kind or another. This leads to confusion about whether the self should be thought of as an object of experience or as a functional unit. Kohut was deliberately ambiguous about definitions of this central element in his theory, at times even praising himself for his ambiguity (1977, pp. 311–312). Many analysts have responded by drawing a distinction between "self" and "self representations." This creates its own problems, especially in light of the many definitions of both terms. Different authors feel called upon to spell out the various connections they see between the self and its representations, and the permutations are endless. Essentially the problem comes down to taking a position on the relation between functioning structures within the mind and our personal, idiosyncratic experience of our mental lives.

I believe that the situation is clarified, and some important ambiguities minimized, if in our theory making we use terms that pointedly lack everyday connotations. So I need a term to indicate clearly that the structure I am proposing is strictly a functional unit of the mind. It is not (and by definition cannot directly become) the object of experience. It can be represented both consciously and unconsciously, but its representations (there are many), like all representations, are not literal renderings. Rather, they are constructions that are multiply determined; a major task of clinical psychoanalysis is to help the analysand deepen his or her understanding of their meaning, origin, and variability. This analytic task is in many ways similar to the exploration of the meaning and origin of the patient's object representations.

Using experience-distant terms in our theorizing can also be helpful clinically. Patients as well as analysts easily confuse personal experience of themselves with the actual condition of underlying mental structures. Many analysands, for example, experience themselves as lacking a cohesive self—since the rise of self psychology this has become something of a badge of honor among the initiated, much as having an Oedipus complex was years ago. Others think of themselves as being "empty" at the core or as having a fundamentally and irredeemably "evil" self. But, in my view, this experience does not reflect any privileged (or "objective") access to the person's actual capabilities, psychopathology, or therapeutic needs.

(See Schafer, 1983, for a similar formulation of the role of personal narrative.) There may well be important discrepancies between experienced defects (multiply determined self representations) and the actual state of underlying structures. The existence and analytic investigation of these discrepancies are highlighted by using structural terms that are experience-distant. The same line of thought persuades me against using other evocative, phenomenologically rich terms such as "I" or "person."

In the end I have chosen to call the central functional unit in my model the *ego*, which I think remains a useful term precisely because it is phenomenologically distant, referring to a functioning structure rather than to an experience. Like any choice, mine brings along its own confusion, because of the traditional use of the term. The major difference between the ego as I conceptualize it and the way the term was used by Freud, and within the ego-psychological emendations of his structural theory, follows from my not finding it useful to retain the structures id and superego in my model. So the ego as I define it is inherently active. It has a directedness that is innate to it, energized by the safety and effectance drives. These drives are not stimuli that impinge upon and activate the ego—they are tendencies that are originally in and always of the ego.

The Construction of Mental Representations

I have argued that in his earliest conflict theory Freud conceptualized the incompatible mental contents as ideas and that these ideas involved different ways of thinking about oneself. Although Freud eventually left this behind, focusing instead on formulations about conflicting forces and on structural conflict, I believe that there was great wisdom in the early vision. It has been brought back into contemporary thinking by a number of analysts, most prominently by Joseph Sandler and George Klein. Both these authors place conflict among different ideas (especially about the self) at the center of their theories of normal development and psychopathology. I find it useful to think of this as conflict among incompatible mental representations.

What are the components of a representation, and how do they become established as contents of the ego? In thinking about this, I begin with the concept of a self representation. I need to be explicit about my reasons for doing so. Because all human experience is cyclical, picking any particular starting point in illustrating a sequence of mental events is necessarily arbitrary and somewhat artificial. Some theorists (especially those operating

within the relational model) would find it more compelling to begin with an interpersonal event. The decision to start with a self representation reflects my own emphasis on the importance of feeling states as regulators of mental activity (Chapter 6). Self representations and feeling states stand in an intimate, reciprocal relationship to each other. The way we are feeling at any moment significantly affects how we imagine ourselves to be (big or small, strong or weak, good or bad). These changing images have been usefully described by Sandler and Rosenblatt (1962) as reflecting changes in the "shape" of the self representation. I will borrow their term throughout my discussion.

The shape of the self representation responds to changing circumstances, both internal and external to the ego. Internal changes include the waxing and waning of safety and effectance needs; external changes derive from the flow of somatic stimuli and from alterations in the person's social situation. External stimuli (including those that arise within the body) are not simply registered passively by the ego; there is always a give and take between perception and motive.

Because self representations are multiply determined constructions, we are capable of thinking about ourselves in many different ways at any moment. Self representations are neither objective nor inevitable, despite patients' frequent claims that they are. We can, however, speak of a particular self representation that dominates experience, both conscious and unconscious. This dominant image has some stability over time, although it is not entirely static.

People form intentions on the basis of their dominant self representations (and their attendant feeling states), which serve as indicators not only of where we are but also of where we would like to go next. Guided by these indicators, we construct wishes, which are themselves represented mentally. The wish has three components: the self, an object, and an interactional field within which the two establish a particular sort of relationship.* The self and object components of the wish are, like all representations, complex and multiply determined. They are drawn from an experience of the need at the moment, from recollected images of self and object under similar conditions of need, and from convictions about the capacities and limits of the self as embodied in its dominant shape.

---

*I owe this formulation to Mitchell's (1988) useful analysis of the components of interpersonal events. I have altered his approach by placing all these components within the subject's experience; that is, I have located all of them as contents of the ego.

Let me illustrate the sequence with a commonplace example from psychoanalytic developmental psychology: the infant's experience of hunger and the psychic and interpersonal events that ensue. The infant's hunger pangs are stimuli external to but impinging upon the ego. Because the subject in my example is an infant, the hunger can be assumed to originate with a somatic stimulus. In the older child or adult, the wish to eat may be equally or primarily instigated by a perceptual or a social stimulus—seeing an advertisement for food or being with a group of people planning a meal. My use of an example from infancy is meant to keep things as simple as possible; but the bodily origin of the stimulus is not essential to an understanding of the process.*

The infant now imagines himself in a particular way; the "hungry self" being fed takes on a specific shape. He will also construct a representation of his mother responding to the hungry self; the "feeding object" has its own shape. The final component of the wish will be a desired exchange between the represented self and the object, one that actualizes the wish to be fed (Sandler, 1981).

The ego attempts to create circumstances in which its wishes can be satisfied, so the infant will initiate an action that is within his capabilities. Since my example is built on the circumstances of the youngest infant, this action is probably limited to crying for the mother. The cry, viewed from this perspective, expresses the infant's active effort to initiate an interpersonal event—to summon the mother and to engage her in the act of feeding (Mahler, 1946). The events set in motion by the cry create the conditions of "perceptual identity" that satisfy the wish (Freud, 1900; Sandler and Sandler, 1978).

We can think of the event initiated by the infant's cry as having the same components as the wish: as the infant participates in it, he will have a particular experience of himself, of the object, and of an interaction between the two. The shapes of the self and the object and the quality of the interaction will have changed from what the infant had imagined when he constructed the original wish. The actual event will only approximate, never duplicate, the original wishful interaction. The infant himself may,

---

*This situation has been considered paradigmatic by psychoanalysts of all theoretical persuasions. It has been used to illustrate (among other things) the process of tension reduction (Rapaport), the role of drive as a nodal point and organizer of a range of relational needs (Jacobson), and the importance of the mother's frame of mind in the infant's experience (Sullivan).

for example, be more or less happy to see his mother when she arrives, and the mother may be more or less happy to be there, depending on her state of mind at the moment. So the interaction between the two is likely to be more or less harmonious, and the various needs that led to the original wish will be more or less satisfied.

I want to be clear about two related sources of potential confusion, both involving the idea of an interaction between the subject and the object. First, because I have described what has occurred as an "event," there may be some implication that there is an actual interaction independent of particular constructions of it. Philosophical conundrums aside, even the simplest interpersonal events are so complex that any notion of "actuality" has to be misleading. My discussion is intended to highlight that the wishing ego is capable of initiating action aimed at satisfying the wish. *Something* has happened because of what the infant has wished; what that something *looks like* will vary from observer to observer.

Second, describing the event as interpersonal may obscure the fact that the event itself may be a fantasy. Again, the description is meant to emphasize the ego's role as agent of events external to it. Fantasies invariably involve such events—among which I include bodily movements and the like. They may also involve the participation of an external object, human or nonhuman, animate or inanimate. But the event may not be noticed (or even noticeable) by anyone other than the person himself. The object of a wishful fantasy may or may not be aware that he or she is participating in it.

In the final step of the process I am describing, the event initiated by the wish is itself mentally represented. Again we have the three familiar components of an event, each multiply determined. The shape of the self is determined by the subject's perception of himself participating in the event, by his experience of the object's perception of him (Sullivan's "reflected appraisals"), and by concurrent bodily and environmental stimuli. *The representation is thus an active construction—in truth a creation—that embodies the event's meaning to the subject.*

The relative impact exerted by the various forces on the shape of the self varies considerably. When bodily stimuli are particularly powerful (extreme sexual excitement is one example, as is intense physical pain), the self representation is organized around them. Similarly, when the interpersonal stimulus conditions are especially compelling (brutal public criticism or enthusiastic support), the reflected appraisals can be the leading

determinants of the representation. Variations in the relative strength of the safety and effectance drives will also play an important role in establishing the shape of the self.

Like the self, the object is a multiply determined construction. It is formed out of the subject's observations of the other (what Freud, 1933, called "impressions"). These reflect the naively perceptual component of the experience of the other, what might be called (if life were not so complex) the "actual" other. Second, there are projections and externalizations, which derive from disowned perceptions of the self as it participated in the event. Perceptions originating in both ways are influenced by the operation and relative strength of the two drives. The processes involved in giving the object its particular shape do not differ in principle from those that determine the shape of the self.

The outcome of any event as it is experienced by the subject alters the shape of both the self and the object representation. When events occur regularly enough to constitute a perceived pattern, these are encoded as a new representational scheme. The components of the scheme include: a self with a certain shape; an object with a certain shape; and an interactional field within which self and object relate to each other in a particular way. The representation of an interactional field calls for particular comment. There are always multiple versions of events and outcomes. Representations, therefore, encode the events as experienced from the subject's particular perspective, which is always one among many.

The Outcome and Representation of Events

Consider the various ways in which the exchange initiated by the hungry infant's wish may be represented. Suppose in the first instance that the infant's wish is unambivalent and that the mother responds to the cry promptly, accurately (by offering food), and lovingly (with appropriate attentiveness and warmth). (In all of what follows we must keep in mind that representations typically develop out of patterns, not discrete events.) Then the child is apt to construct the components of a representation along these lines:

1. His needs themselves are good, because they lead to gratifying experiences. (Sullivan, 1953, probably had this in mind when he thought of needs as "integrating tendencies.")

2. He is an effective executive of his needs, because he is able to create the conditions of gratification. (Winnicott, 1960, p. 146, addressed this

aspect of the development of the self when he spoke of the "illusion of omnipotent creating" that accompanies the satisfaction of needs.)

3. He is a member in good standing of the human community, because other important people value and support his needs.

4. His mother, in her own right, is a strong and giving person, capable of understanding and delivering what he needs—she is someone who can be counted on.

5. Experienced interactions can approximate wishful fantasies. Satisfaction can be achieved with no damage to either participant.

These impressions (which even in somebody much older than the infant of our example may or may not be conscious and most likely cannot be given verbal expression) determine the shapes of the self, object, and interactional field as they were experienced in the course of the lived event. They become the stuff of a new representation. It is a function of the ego to store the representations it has constructed, and this addition becomes a new mental content.

The new representation, as a component of the person's life experience, will become a significant determinant of the person's feeling state and of his dominant self representation. The event (as experienced and represented) influences the feeling state, but the feeling state also influences the experience of the event itself. The feeling state indicates whether the event has achieved its desired result (fulfillment of the wish) or whether things have taken a different turn (generating anxiety, depression, or some other unpleasant affect) so that action needs to be aborted. The feeling state provides "terminal feedback" (G. Klein, 1967) for the action initiated by the wish.

Through its influence on the feeling state and the dominant shape of the self, the new representation will be a stimulus to subsequent wishes. The event in my example had a favorable outcome, with positively valued representations of both self and object. Accordingly, the infant will most likely want more contact with his mother or with other people; or he may wish for more stimuli that motivate activity, because he anticipates that the sequence of need-action-event is reliable and will be satisfying. At the same time, the infant's sense of his own effectiveness takes some of the urgency out of his need for others; he will learn to trust and to value his potential as an autonomous individual. Successful experiences of this sort contribute both to optimism about relations with others and to what Winnicott called "the capacity to be alone" (1958).

The lived event and its stored representation will also be associated with

specific affective states.* In the example, the evoked affects will reflect the experienced well-being and collaboration of self and object. Affects associated with these representations include warmth, trust, love, and so on. The affective valence of a representation is particularly important because it is a major factor in the subject's organization of experience; representations cluster together when they have similar emotional tones. In Chapter 8 I will emphasize that affect is also decisively associated with the accessibility to consciousness of representations.

IN MY discussion so far I have confined myself to the processes involved in the representation and fulfillment of a hypothetically unambivalent wish. There can be two wrinkles. In the first, the infant is still hungry and the mother again responds promptly, accurately, and lovingly. But the child is also feeling a particular need to act autonomously and at a distance from his mother. This need may originate from any one of a number of sources: innate fluctuations in the drives; the impact of specific interpersonal stimuli; or the feedback from a represented experience Whatever the source, though, the child is in conflict about what he wants to do or to have happen next. So no event can be fully satisfying. The mother's empathy itself—her appreciation of the infant's hunger and her response to it—breaches the emotional space between them that he also wants to preserve; this frustrates his wish for autonomy and distance. Preserving the distance, on the other hand, would necessarily leave the child hungry.

The child's ambivalence—still at a level that is well within the "normal" range and that may in fact be normative—will affect the quality of the actual interpersonal event and especially the characteristics of its representation. In contrast to what was represented in the first example:

1. His needs are not as unequivocally good as they were in the first example, because their satisfaction brings along with it an unwelcome, even threatening impingement.

2. His own sense of agency is likely to be compromised, because he is unable to satisfy needs that are (from an outsider's perspective, although

---

*The limitations of psychoanalytic conceptions of affect are widely lamented. This is only partially justified. By all accounts, affective states have significant neurophysiological determinants: it is reasonable to assume that to some extent affect reflects bodily changes and enters psychological experience as an innate determinant rather than an effect of lived experience (Kernberg, 1982). Psychoanalysis, then, is not able to offer a comprehensive theory of affect. The scheme I develop here refers to affect only as it arises as a reaction to the outcome of events and becomes a significant component of their representation.

most likely not from the infant's own) inherently conflictual. Unaware of his dilemma directly, the child experiences himself as less capable.

3. Partly because she must actually fail to meet the child's needs in these circumstances, and partly as a result of the child's externalization of his own sense of failure and of having been impinged upon, the mother is experienced as unsatisfying and as presenting the danger of crushing the child's strivings for autonomy.

These altered circumstances influence the shape of all elements of the represented event. Because the child could neither satisfy his needs nor ward off his mother's "intrusion," he felt helpless and impinged upon. The self will be represented as needy (perhaps more urgently needy than at the beginning of the event), but also as weak and ineffective. In contrast, the mother will be represented as overly powerful and intrusive. This impression is likely to be magnified by the child's externalization of his anger with himself for being incapable of meeting his own needs. Rage and contempt will be projected, and will become an important component of the object representation.*

The affects generally associated with this configuration of self and object are humiliation, envy, and fearful hatred. The extent to which these are actually evoked will depend on the intensity of the underlying conflict and on the mother's ability to perceive it and adjust herself accordingly—by maintaining an emotional distance while feeding, for example. Let me stress, however, that there is no "optimal" or fully corrective response to conflicted wishes.

The feeling state generated by this event and its dominant self representation will be strikingly different than in my first example. The child will not simply seek more contact, either with the mother or with any other person. In benign circumstances it may move the developing infant to imagine feeding himself, thus to experiment with newly emerging capabilities in the service of individuation. Less fortuitously, it may evoke wishes to withdraw when under the pressure of need or to engage the mother in a more submissive way. The outcome in any particular case will be influenced by many factors, notably including the relative strength of

---

*I plead guilty to some mixing of metaphors here. I picked an infant for my example out of a wish to keep things simple from a motivational standpoint. But the infant is surely not capable of the complex cognitive operations I describe. Although there is something fictive in the example, the capacities do begin early in childhood. There is value as well in assuming genetic continuity dating to the very beginning, and so it makes sense to talk about some rudimentary version of the process going on from the start of life.

the safety and effectance drives. A range of such events, and the establishment of their representations, is part and parcel of normal development.

In this example, the experienced outcome of event and its representation had very little to do with the actual exchange or with the actions of the mother. Rather, they were determined by the qualities of the child's motivational state. In other circumstances, complications arise not because of the child's wish but as a result of his mother's response. Assume that the child is hungry and that the wish to be fed is not significantly marked by conflicting needs. But his mother, who has been having a particularly bad day, feels imposed upon and responds to his need less eagerly than she usually does—although still, as in my previous example, well within the normal fluctuations of everyday life.* She feeds the child, but without her usual enthusiasm for the encounter; she wishes that he weren't hungry again and would just go to sleep. As the feeding continues, she wants it to go faster. She feels (and acts) depleted.

In this example, an "environmental" problem affects the interpersonal event and its representation. Again, both self and object representations will be influenced:

1. The child will feel that his needs are bad, not because they endanger him but because they endanger the object. He believes that he cannot be a trusted member of society because he wants too much or wants the wrong things.

2. His sense of agency again is compromised, because he can satisfy himself only by victimizing somebody else. He can be powerful, but his power is hurtful.

3. He experiences his mother as weak, destructible, perhaps even at his mercy. This impression is based upon the child's observation of his mother's experience of imposition and depletion in the face of his needs.

So the child experiences himself as having satisfied a specific need, his hunger, but at his mother's expense. In his mind he has remained intact (and has even gained what he wants); his mother has crumbled. The evoked shapes of self and object reflect this outcome: an unrestrained and unrelenting self is engaged with a weakened object. As always, projective and introjective processes as well as the actual interpersonal event influence

---

*This hypothetical situation is similar to one posited by Sullivan (1953) in which the child's hunger is met by a mother who is ready and able to feed him, but who is anxious for reasons that may have nothing to do with the child. I depart from Sullivan in not restricting the source of disturbance to the specific affect of anxiety. In contrast I believe that many states of mind can interfere with the interpersonal event.

these representations. The mother may be acting tired, for example, but the representation of her as depleted is partially drawn from the child's self experience, including the experience of his failure to engage his mother fully in the current exchange. Similarly, his sense of himself as brutally strong has an introjective component; in the represented event the mother is also brutal in her failure to respond in accord with the child's wishes.

The affective consequences of this sort of exchange reflect the child's experience of having damaged his mother in pursuit of his own satisfaction. Typically, this leads to feelings of guilt and remorse, which will characterize the event as it is represented.

Feedback from the representation of this event will contribute to a feeling state and a dominant self representation that reflect the child's belief in his destructiveness. This will not lead to wishes for similar sorts of contact with another person. Instead there will be pressure to avoid the destructive effects of such powerful needs. Wishes constructed under the influence of this feedback may, consequently, represent a weaker, less competent, regressed self in interaction with an object that is strengthened by contrast with the child's passivity. Or the wishes may conceive a self without any needs at all, passively guided by the preferences of others, who are thereby protected from potential assault. In other circumstances, the representation may be one source of future sadistic wishes. It can become the core of the ruthlessness that Winnicott sees as part of the child's innate endowment—but I believe it develops as the result of early relational experience.

Triangular Events

So far I have addressed only wishes and events involving two people. In the course of development, however, the dyad increasingly and inexorably becomes a fiction. Quickly the child is a member of a family; he is enmeshed in a social network. Generally I don't think psychoanalytic theory takes this change in the nature of experience seriously enough. As Freud first conceived it, the triangulation of the Oedipus complex brought the father into the child's psychological universe for the first time, introducing some new emotions—jealousy, rivalry, guilt, and the like. But this formulation has not held up well in the light of subsequent investigation. The father appears on the scene much earlier than Freud imagined, and the young child's affects have a greater range than he thought possible. Many of the psychological characteristics originally attributed to triangu-

lar relationships are demonstrable in the dyadic period, so triangulation itself has lost much of its meaning.

I think it is crucial, both theoretically and clinically, to restore triangular relationships to the center stage of psychoanalytic thought. That is why in my opening chapter I addressed the centrality of the Oedipus complex in my psychoanalytic vision. We are now in a position to go further with the discussion. The psychological difference between dyadic and triangular relationships does not depend merely on the number of people involved: the distinction is that in triangular relationships the subject has a sense (consciously or unconsciously) that the events in which he is involved have consequences beyond the immediate situation. Most triangular events occur in the physical presence of only two people. But, when the child becomes capable of triangular experience, *there is always a relationship with the person who is not there.*

This is clear in the oedipal situation, the prototype of triangular relationships in the same sense that the hungry infant and his mother is the prototype of the dyad. The boy alone with his mother knows that what goes on between the two of them (significantly including the child's fantasies) has an impact on his father. It will affect not only the reciprocal attitudes between father and son (jealousy, rivalry, guilt), but also the way the mother feels about her husband and the way the father feels about his wife. The oedipal child knows that he is at the center of a reverberating system of interpersonal events.

Triangulation thus signals the subject's initiation into a social network of which he is an effective member—a process that has been well described by Loewald (1979) and, from quite a different perspective, by Ogden (1989). In this sense, the term itself is somewhat misleading. The psychological significance of triangular relationships lies in the representation of a social network; the triad embodies not just a third person but all those not immediately present. Narrowly equating the triad with the third person has kept analysts since Freud from fully exploring the psychodynamic role of relationships with siblings, grandparents, members of the extended family, and the community at large.

The advent of triangular wishes, events, and their representation both depends upon and facilitates developments in the cognitive equipment that the ego has at its disposal. On the one hand, the subject must be able to imagine effects that operate across spatial and temporal distance. On the other, beginning awareness that there are such effects motivates the subject to use and improve his imaginative capacities. This process can

often be observed in the course of psychoanalytic work with adults; it can be presumed to operate analogously in the course of early development.

Consider the sequence involved in the formation of a wish, the initiation of an interpersonal event, and the representation of the event. The process begins with a feeling state part of which is a dominant self representation. But from the outset the wish born out of the feeling state is triangulated. A third person is psychologically present for the subject, although the subject himself may be thoroughly unconscious of that presence.

As in my discussion of dyadic experience, wishes lead to particular sorts of interaction with the subject's immediate object. In addition, however, pursuit of the wish inevitably creates a relationship with a third person. The third person—actually the multiply determined representation that is a creation of the subject's ego—has feelings about the subject's pursuit of the wish. These feelings reflect attitudes about the subject himself, about the object of the wish, or about the kind of activity involved in fulfilling the wish. The nature of the wish itself is an important determinant of the shape of the representation of the absent third person.

This is in line with Freud's idea that the boy's image of a punitive oedipal father varies according to the strength of the child's own incestuous wishes. It broadens that formulation, however, by including other perceptual and motivational forces among the determinants of the representation. Freud focused on the child's hostility and fear; I would include equally his love, concern, loyalty, identifications, impressions, and so on.

Consider how this formulation illuminates what happens when an oedipal boy imagines making more or less direct sexual overtures to his mother. Typically the third person involved will be the boy's father. The father will (in the boy's experience) have feelings about the boy, for instance love, rivalry, identifications, jealousy, or paternal hopes. He will also have feelings about his wife, attachment to her, possessiveness, or admiration and respect. Finally, he will have feelings about the boy's particular aims—perhaps an attraction to or a fear of phallic expression, perhaps an attraction to or fear of aggressive/possessive attitudes toward women.

From all these particulars, the boy will construct a representation of his father's attitude toward the oedipal wish and of the relationship with his father that pursuing the wish will involve. This gives the representation of the third person a particular shape and defines the represented interaction between this person and the subject.

Triangulation also involves representation of an interaction between the

third person and the object of the wish. It is part of the definition of triangulation as I am discussing it that the subject has some experience of the effects of his wishes on distant events. The oedipal boy imagines that his wishes affect the relationship between his mother and father. He may come to believe that the wishes drive his parents apart. Perhaps he believes that the mother prefers him and gets more pleasure from his advances than from his father's. Perhaps she uses his wish as an occasion to withdraw from or to take some revenge against the father. In other circumstances the child may sense that his wishes bring his parents closer together. He may pose a threat to their own secure dyad or to their own oedipal solutions. So they unite in order to exclude and punish him for wanting what is forbidden.

The representations of triangular experiences are vastly more complicated than those of dyadic relationships. The nature of the wish affects and is affected by the subject's representation of his relationship with the third person, and his idea of the relationship between the third person and the object of the wish. One consequence is that the interaction between subject and object is deformed by the influence of the third person. If the third person is hostile or vulnerable to actualization of the wished-for interaction, this may manifest itself as an indirect satisfaction of the wish (through aim inhibition, relegation to fantasy, displacement, or some other defensive activity). On the other hand, the third person may have a particular stake in the subject's pursuing the activity. An inhibited father may, for example, relish his son's free expression of phallic aggression. The boy will then enact the role of oedipal conquistador, perhaps with more bravado than he comfortably feels.

When an experience instigated by a triangulated wish is represented, all components of the representation are affected. The experience has consequences not only for the shapes of self, object, and third person, but also for the representations of the relationships among all three people. The boy's experience of his oedipally driven exchange with his mother includes ideas about his relationship with his father, and about the quality of his father's continuing relationship with his mother.

My formulation so far casts light on the pivotal role that triangular experience plays in psychoanalytic construction. It points to the intimate relation between triangulation and the dynamic centrality of agency, conflict, and fantasy. Let me sketch this relation, beginning with the last.

Fantasy. Triangulated experience almost always involves relationships with a person who is not present. In addition, it includes a relationship—

between the object and the absent third person—the details of which are at best partially accessible to the subject. The child gets only glimpses of what goes on between his parents. About the rest he is necessarily left to wonder.

This contrasts markedly with the quality of dyadic experience. Because dyadic experience typically involves a present and participating object, its representation is significantly influenced by the object's actual behavior. Although representations are always idiosyncratic, the subject's observations play a major role. The angry, hungry child may fantasize destroying his mother's breast in the act of sucking, and this may become an important aspect of his represented interaction with his mother. But at the same time, the mother's continuing presence reassures the child and limits the influence of the destructive fantasy and its attendant fears. The corrective potential of actual interpersonal exchanges is a keystone of Melanie Klein's understanding of the origin and development of object relations. It is also an aspect of Daniel Stern's suggestion that the very young infant is "an excellent reality-tester" (1985, p. 11).

In contrast, triangular experience does not permit this sort of correction. Because one participant in the exchange is absent, events are set in motion that remain inaccessible to the subject's observation. What cannot be directly perceived is constructed and elaborated upon by the imaginings of the subject. He will imagine how his exchange with the object affects the third person, how this will influence his current and future relationship with that person, and how the relationship between the object and the third person will be influenced. The oedipal boy, for example, must imagine what effect his sexual overtures to his mother have on his relationship with his father or on the relationship between the two parents.

Eventually, of course, the child has a chance to observe his father and to see how his parents act toward each other. But this is likely to happen some time after the original event. The vast terra incognita that characterizes triangular experience greatly increases the impact that fantasy has on the entire sequence. The wish itself is shaped by fantasies about the third person's relationship with both self and object. The interaction with the object in turn is deformed by fantasies about the third person. Finally, there are multiply determined representations of self, object, and third person which are significantly determined by fantasied effects that elude correction. For this reason, the effects of fantasies will be encoded and fixed as an essential component of the represented experience.

Conflict. I have argued throughout that conflict is inherent in human experience as constructed by the psychoanalytic method and that, because of the tension between the safety and effectance drives, some degree of conflict can be presumed active from the beginning of life. Both the ubiquity and the importance of conflict are even more evident when relationships are triangular. Consider the nature of the attachment that the subject has to the third person. He will experience the complex mix of feelings—concern, loyalty, fear, love, hostility—that characterize intimate relationships. Because the experience is triangular, the wished-for interaction with the object affects relations with the third person that are motivated by these feelings. Triangular experience can be unconflicted only if there is perfect attunement among the people involved. This can never happen, so there will always be some conflict of interpersonal origin. Equally important, because triangular experience is always fantastically elaborated, the characteristics of the represented objects are significantly inferential. The oedipal child who believes that his attachment to his mother means that his father will feel betrayed and damaged may well believe it irrespective of how his father actually feels or acts. There still is wisdom in Freud's insistence that the oedipal father is a construction based on the child's wishes.

Agency. I have defined the ego as an inherently active structure in order to emphasize the presumption of agency intrinsic in all human behavior and experience. Like conflict, however, the subject's contribution to experience is more evident in triangular events. This follows from the discussion of fantasy and conflict.

The place that fantasy has in the construction of triangulated wishes suggests that from the beginning of the sequence I have described the subject is actively shaping his inner world. To the extent that representations do not simply mirror externally derived impressions, we can see how the subject creates his mental contents and is the agent of his experience.

The role of agency is also highlighted when we appreciate that conflicting pressures lie behind all actions. Every triangulated wish involves both an impression of and an interest in the object and the third person. The subject chooses among these interests, which are inevitably at odds with one another to some degree. A different way of putting this is to say that triangulated wishes always involve alternatives (in terms of desires, attachments, loyalties, fears). Alternatives require choice, and choice implies agency.

Repression

THE MODEL I have begun to develop can contribute significantly to our thinking about the dynamic relationship among mental representations, and thus to our understanding of the clinically crucial problem of repression. But, to repeat, the problem itself is vexing. How does it happen that some mental contents are so aversive that we sacrifice the pursuit of urgent personal goals, self-knowledge, and acuity about others in the service of remaining unaware of them? I will begin my discussion with a vignette, not strictly clinical but human.

A child at the age of about a year and a half develops a special taste for lima beans. She requests them frequently, reacts gleefully when they arrive, and asks for extra portions. When mixed vegetables are served the first thing she does is to go through the pile and pick out all the lima beans, setting them apart and eating them with obvious pleasure. She asks others to pick out their lima beans and give them to her, and she is excited and grateful when they do.

This goes on for a year or so. Gradually the child's enthusiasm for the lima beans wanes. She asks for them less frequently and doesn't pick them out from the mixed vegetables. Lima beans are no longer a center of attention at mealtimes, either for her or for her family.

Time passes and one day the girl, now three years old, once again goes through her mixed vegetables and picks out all the lima beans. She sets them aside and eats everything else. Her surprised parents ask her about it. "I hate lima beans," she answers. "You used to love them," they say. "No I didn't," replies the girl, "I hate them and I've always hated them." Not yet catching on to the intensity of the child's feeling, the parents press on. "Don't you remember when you used to pick them out of the pile and eat

them first, and ask for everybody else's?" The child becomes visibly upset: "No I didn't. I hate them, and I hate you too!" Her parents acknowledge that maybe they were wrong, the subject is dropped, and things get back on an even keel within a few minutes.

In this example we can see the effects of repression, complete with the anxiety and secondary defenses that frequently accompany the return of the repressed. The child's reaction is reminiscent of the way analytic patients sometimes respond to accurate but poorly timed or heavy-handed interpretations. Both her tenacious denial and her anger suggest that there is something there, that her parents' comments have rung some sort of bell, but that it is not something that she wants to be forcibly reminded of, at least not at the moment.

Why did the child turn her back on lima beans? Was there some conflict that required her to renounce the old object of her affections? It is probably reasonable to guess that at the beginning there was neither conflict nor repression. Tastes change, and passions wane. Our connections with things, interests, and people are constantly in a state of flux. The child lost her taste for lima beans—nobody really knows why, except that such changes are part of the normal ebbs and flows of life. But this does not account for what happened at the dinner table. It fails to explain either the tenacity with which the child denied her former love or the intensity of her emotions. By the time things heated up, the child was clearly in conflict—a conflict that was interpersonalized in the struggle between her and her parents. At the dinner table there *was* repression; whatever memories of having once loved lima beans the child had were vigorously kept out of conscious awareness. To understand how this came about, we have to go beyond what I said about changing interests.

Our involvements with things, interests, and people are central to the way we think about ourselves, as we are in the present and as we were in the past. These involvements are the stuff of mental representations, and the individual elements of the representation have enormous evocative power. A briefly recalled image of something we once cared about transports us to another place and time, when both we and the world were very different. We have all had the experience with a snippet of melody; couples hearing "our song" from many years ago become young again. Proust's *madeleine* is an icon etched in our cultural consciousness.

For the child in my example, being reminded that she once loved lima beans—a love that she no longer felt—evoked the feeling of being a much

younger child. This feeling threatened her sense of having grown and matured, of having *outgrown* the earlier pleasure. It is at this point that we can first speak of a potential or emergent conflict. On one side was her sense of herself as progressing, moving forward, becoming more competent and powerful. On the other side was a regressive pull back to an earlier self, one that had experienced pleasures in its own way but represents an abandonment of what she has achieved. This conflict, intensified and pushed toward consciousness by her parents' inquiry, made it painful to accept their reminder of her early love of lima beans. The love was too evocative, too closely associated with a now intolerable self-image.

Being confronted with her earlier passion left the child feeling ashamed and humiliated; these are the affective concomitants of believing oneself incompetent. Both her anxiety and the urgency of her defensive operations increased: she warded off awareness more tenaciously and became increasingly projective. This is a commonplace sequence in psychological development, in the course of psychoanalytic treatment, and in everyday life. Consider the contempt that children of a certain age have for their "babyish" juniors. They feel similarly about their own self representations. Nostalgia is a pleasure only when one feels safely able to resist the pull of regression.

I have skewed my example for simplicity's sake. In particular I have focused exclusively on the child's endogenous motives for repressing an earlier self representation: thinking of herself as loving lima beans (and loving them as she did at a year and a half) is incompatible with her contemporary developmental needs, which include seeing herself in a more "grown-up" way. Of course this is an incomplete picture, because it sets aside interpersonal contributions. We cannot fully understand what happened unless we know more about the parents' attitudes toward regressive tendencies (in the child and in themselves). The child's reaction to thinking of herself as younger than she actually is—how tolerant she is of the ebbs and flows of developmental advance and retreat—are significantly shaped by these attitudes. Similarly, the parents' feelings about things they love and once loved influence the way the child relates to these images of herself. And do her parents share attitudes toward these issues or do they feel very differently about them, so that the child's reactions move her toward one parent and away from the other? Whatever the actual facts, the child's various self representations are likely to evoke a range of identifications and qualities of relatedness with both parents, which in turn

will influence what she can and cannot experience consciously. Add a sibling (either younger or older) to the mix and the possibilities ramify even more.

But however we understand the elements of the child's conflict, the vignette supports a view of repression that guided Freud's early thinking (both clinical and theoretical) and that has reemerged in the writings of Kohut, George Klein, and Sandler: people need to keep certain mental contents out of consciousness because these contents evoke intolerably painful self representations. The pain arises when there is an intensely felt discrepancy between the dominant self representation and others that threaten to enter awareness. Psychic conflict intense enough to instigate repression originates with the incompatibility of various "shapes" of the self. Repression safeguards the integrity of the self.

Repression of Wishes

Consider the steps involved in forming a mental representation as I described them in Chapter 7. The process begins with a feeling state embodied in an image of the self with a particular shape, then moves to a wish, then to an event undertaken to satisfy the wish, and concludes with a representation of the event. Repression may be directed either at the wish or at the representation of the event instigated by the wish.* The only difference between a repressed wish and a conscious one, or between a repressed representation and a conscious one is accessibility to awareness (Freud, 1915b, p. 149). People initiate actions on the basis of unconscious wishes, and banished representations continue to color experience. The motive for repression is the same whether the intolerable mental content is a wish or a representation, but the steps involved are somewhat different.

Wishes are formed out of the convergence of a number of determinants: the ebbs and flows of safety and effectance needs; perceived external circumstances including but not limited to perceptions of somatic and interpersonal stimuli; and the representations of events initiated by recent

---

*I am using the concept of repression broadly, to describe the process by which we banish all sorts of mental contents from awareness, observations of what goes on around us as well as wishes that arise endogenously. In putting things like this I am in agreement with Dorpat (1985), who argues persuasively that one "basic defense" controls access to consciousness of both internally and externally derived contents. Dorpat calls this basic defense denial, but I prefer repression, which has always been central in psychoanalytic theory and practice.

wishes. The wish contains a representation of the self with a particular shape. This represented self may be quite similar to the shape of the self that is dominant in consciousness when the wish is formed, but it may also be quite different. Recall that this dominant self representation is itself subject to change in accord with changing internal and external conditions.

Whether the wish can become conscious depends on the degree of compatibility between the shape of the dominant self representation and the shape of the self in the wish. The wish itself may be sexual, dependent, destructive, ambitious, or anything else. Its content is more or less irrelevant; what matters is how people envision themselves when they imagine pursuing the wish. *Any* wish will be repressed if it contains a self representation too disharmonious with what is acceptable at the moment (see G. Klein, 1976, p. 186).

Consider this clinical illustration of both the repression of a wish and the continuing impact that the wish exerts on behavior and experience. A patient who has struggled mightily with conflicts over her professional ambitions gets a job offer that has good possibilities for advancement. Characteristically, she cannot acknowledge that she has successfully pursued a possibility; she insists it is merely something that inadvertently (and perhaps even mistakenly) happened to her. She is taking a while to make up her mind about the offer. When she talks about it, she focuses on the burden and responsibility that would be involved. She insists that she's not good enough, that she would disappoint her superiors and would soon feel depressed and overwhelmed. She says nothing about *wanting* the job and certainly nothing about feeling flattered or enthusiastic or excited about the offer. Her mood in the sessions reflects these feelings: she seems depressed, passive, unproductive, unreflective.

Within a few days of making her decision, the patient reports several events, which she sees as unrelated to the new opportunity. She was publicly criticized by colleagues at work for being arrogant and insensitive. Then she got into a dispute with a man who supplies some important professional equipment; if her relationship with this man is disrupted, her new plans may be jeopardized. And she made some more than characteristically demanding sexual advances to her husband on a night when he didn't feel well, leading him to accuse her of hostility and self-centeredness. As a result of each exchange, the patient feels deflated, degraded, and weakened. These self representations are enacted in her behavior in the analysis.

It took some work before we could get beyond these thoughts and actions to a deeper understanding of the sequence that began with the job offer. The offer had in fact excited the patient. She had begun to see herself in the new position, commanding attention, wielding power, feeling and being attractive in a markedly potent way. Moreover, in her most private moments, she had embarrassedly thrilled at the idea; it would feel not only good, but right. The excitement also affected her transference feelings; in this frame of mind her relationship to me looked quite different. Now she was a challenge, a threat, and a seductress. Both sexually and professionally she would have to cope differently with me, and I with her. She could no longer be the little girl in thrall to a powerful mentor/protector.

It was the wish organized around this excited, exciting self representation that the patient could not tolerate in consciousness. For a variety of reasons based in her history, but not essential to the example at this point, that self representation had become incompatible with a dominant view of herself as incompetent, passive, needy, asexual, and above all harmless. Whenever she was "plagued by" wishes like the one just described (that was her experience, not my interpretation), she was especially tenacious in her attempts to repress them. She had developed an impressive array of secondary defenses, generally involving interpersonal enactments. These forced upon her (again, her characterization) the experience of a defeated, degraded self that, although consciously unpleasant, felt safe and familiar.

It was these secondary defenses that were played out in the events my patient described after receiving the job offer. She managed to induce others to react to her in a way that strikingly reflected her own judgment of the ambitious, powerful, excited self represented in the wish. They told her that she was pushy, aggressive, arrogant, inconsiderate, selfish, and exhibitionistic. The meaning of such comments for the patient was that she was destructively messy, like a child who soils herself with excrement or an adolescent who appears in public with stains of menstrual blood on her clothes. Both images had ample meaning in her own life experience. People's reactions, which she played a significant role in inducing, reinforced the patient's fears of what being ambitious or exciting meant about her. Thus they reinforced the repression of the wish and also helped to sustain the dominant self representations.

Repression of Representations

I will begin this discussion with a commonplace observation about child development. Educators unanimously agree that reading to children fre-

quently when they are very young will encourage them to develop a love of reading later on. Parents are advised to read to their children every day to prepare them for learning to read themselves. The observation makes sense intuitively. There can be a great feeling of warmth, sharing, and involvement when parents read aloud. Reading together becomes a high point of the day, infused with a powerful sense of intimacy.

The educators' advice works: children exposed to this experience do tend to develop a love of reading on their own. But strikingly, once they learn how to read, these children (at least for a very long time) do not want to be read to. In fact, they may make it quite clear that they deeply resent their parents for wanting to read aloud. They want to read by themselves, and if reading is going to be a group activity at all, they insist on being the one who reads to others.

This development defies easy understanding. Clearly the early events have influenced the child's subsequent experience. Things would have turned out differently had there been no reading by the parents. But why doesn't the child want to repeat these earlier sources of pleasure? Intuition says that what has been good should continue to be good and should be sought after. But the child who has learned to read finds the previously enjoyable experience highly aversive.

We are left with this: once the child has learned how to read, being reminded that he once enjoyed being read to is painful. The child reacts to recollections of an old pleasure (much as the young lima-bean lover did) as if it were an assault on his competence or a seduction into passivity, as if he were being seen as younger than he really is. This will be especially true until the new skill (and the child's sense of himself as possessing it) is firmly consolidated.

In terms of a representational model, we can put it this way: when the child was younger, the experience of being read to was infused with good feelings. The child saw himself as a valued and powerful member of the family, capable and worthy of taking part in an activity that gave pleasure both to himself and to others. He felt competent because he participated fully in the activity, in a way that was appropriate to his age and abilities. This meant listening to the story, asking or answering questions about the pictures, naming the letters, responding alertly and with interest. The shapes of the self representations derived from the events reflect this experience. The child is a valuable and valued partner in a lively and enjoyable undertaking.

The decisive change is achieving a new ability. Learning how to read dramatically affects not only the contemporary self representation but also

the child's attitude toward the earlier one. With the acquisition of this very important new skill, the memories of being read to no longer look the same. The child can only experience a not-yet-able-to-read self (his own or anybody else's) as weak and babyish. Now the child shuns his old pleasure. He refuses to be read to and perhaps even leaves the room when others are reading aloud. But the change goes even deeper, because the child is not even able to recall how good being read to once felt. This suggests that once the new skill is acquired, the shape of the self in recollected experiences of being read to undergoes a retrospective change. I will call the process leading to this change *re-representation*.

Quite early on, Freud noticed something similar to what I am describing. Succinctly characterizing memory as "tendentious," he alluded to an interesting aspect of the problem in his paper on "Screen Memories":

> In the majority of significant and in other respects unimpeachable childhood scenes the subject sees himself in the recollection as a child, with the knowledge that this child is himself; he sees this child, however, as an observer from outside the scene would see him . . . Now it is evident that such a picture cannot be an exact repetition of the impression that was originally received. For the subject was then in the middle of the situation and was attending not to himself but to the external world (1899, p. 321).

On the basis of this observation, Freud reached a conclusion that was stunning at the time and remains suggestive today:

> Our childhood memories show us our earliest years not as they were but as they appeared at the later periods when the memories were aroused. In these periods of arousal, the childhood memories did not, as people are accustomed to say, *emerge;* they were *formed* at that time. And a number of motives, with no concern for historical accuracy, had a part in forming them, as well as in the selection of the memories themselves (p. 322).

Unfortunately, Freud's theoretical commitments led him to explain these inaccuracies of memory in a way that kept him from following through the implications of his remarks. The recollected events, he said, were constructed to screen the existence of forbidden fantasies. The fantasies, not the memories themselves, threaten psychic equilibrium. This is another example of how psychoanalytic attention was diverted from the event (which became a mere screen) to the impulse.*

---

*In an early analogy, Freud caught something of the perspective I am proposing. The falsification of childhood memory, he suggested, is similar to the way nations rewrite their history to support "present beliefs and wishes" (1910a, p. 83; also 1901, p. 48). But the

A representational perspective offers a different, and I think more satisfying, explanation of what Freud described. The process begins with the
subject involved in some kind of event. Although it may help to envision
this as an event occurring between two (or possibly more) people, it is not
necessarily interpersonal. There could be something going on between the
subject and an external object, but there needn't be (and perhaps generally
isn't) anybody else directly involved. It could be something that the subject observes (an exchange between other people, a play or movie, a song,
Proust's *madeleine*). It could be a purely internal fantasy or even simply a
nostalgic mood. Frequently it is a wish for some abandoned earlier source
of pleasure. In any case, the importance of the event in this instance is that
it instigates the recall of some earlier representation.

This process of recall happens as it does because of the way that representations are stored. To understand this, we must go back to the construction of the representation itself. When a particular sort of experience
has reached a threshold level of psychological importance (because it has
occurred frequently or because it has been particularly intense), a representation of it is constructed. Once established, representations never disappear (Sandler and Rosenblatt, 1962; Sandler and Sandler, 1987). They
are stored permanently, but not randomly. Representations cluster in patterns determined by various sorts of associative links.

The problem of links among elements stored in memory has been addressed more by cognitive psychologists than by psychoanalysts. Attempting to bridge the gap between the two perspectives, Morris Eagle has
arrived at a conclusion rather similar to mine. Memories, he writes, are
"stored as sets of features, any one or more of which can be selectively
activated and 'appear' in recall." These activated schemata can be linked to
other schemata in a variety of ways (1987, p. 165). Drawing on the data
of cognitive psychology, Eagle points to theories about the way words are
stored as collections of different features: their first letter, number of syl-
lables, the superordinate category to which they belong. This would account for being able to remember the first letter of a word that is on the
tip of one's tongue or recalling a word that is associatively linked to a word
one is groping for.

In the clinical psychoanalytic model I am proposing, the different com-

---

power of the drive model undercut this idea. Eventually Freud came to believe that if the
distorting, drive-derived fantasies can be made conscious, the historically true memory will
become accessible. This was certainly his view when he was making elaborate constructions
in the Wolf Man case (1918).

ponents of a represented event provide the links. The storage system (in agreement with Eagle's cognitive formulation) is typically unconscious. Only a small fraction of the representations and virtually none of the connections among them are in awareness at any particular time. Some common links include similarities among shapes of the self representation; shapes of the object representation; qualities of the interactional field; the balance of drive derived needs that contributed to the particular characteristics of the interaction; the nature of any external (somatic or environmental) stimuli that played a role; and the quality of the feeling state that infuses the whole experience. The evocation of old representations is constant, the natural result of their clustering on the basis of multiple associative links.

Even when evoked, the old representations themselves do not become conscious. What we get is a moment, more or less ephemeral, more or less on the fringes of awareness, when we feel something similar to what we felt at the time of the original represented event. We get a glimmer of the old experience of ourselves, perhaps loving something in the way we once loved it—in my examples so far, being read to or being thrilled by the special pile of lima beans. What enters awareness at these moments is a kind of emotional reverberation; the representation itself is dynamically active, but not conscious.

Our reactions to old representations depend not only on the the nature of the early experience itself, but also on the state of the dominant self representation. Consider the child who has just learned how to read. If he is secure in his new capacity and comfortable with himself as a reader, the old representations can enrich his experience of the new activity. Although they remain unconscious, they become an important source of the pleasure that accompanies the child's own reading. In reading *by* himself the child is also reading *to* himself, and the unconscious reverberation of old pleasures deepens the meaning of the experience and gives it a special poignance. This will be intense years later, when the child, grown now, reads to his own children. The identification with the child is powerful enough that, if by now he is comfortable enough about being grown-up, he will almost consciously experience a paradoxical feeling of reading and being read to at the same time.

But the situation is very different when the dominant self representation is less dependably established. Let me apply the scheme to the child who has just learned to read. He has become an avid reader; he spends a good deal of his time reading and doing things connected to reading. The dom-

inant self representation is significantly shaped by his new ability to read and by his feelings about himself for possessing that competence. He also has strong feelings about people (including his earlier self) who do not possess it. But the child has not been a reader for long; he is not fully certain of his ability to resist the dangers (and temptations) of regression.

Let us suppose that something has happened in this child's life to evoke a representation of being read to. Perhaps it's simply that his parents suggested that they read to him, or perhaps on his own he has had the impulse to be read to. The evoked representation (the image of being read to) is unconscious. It is, however, resonating affectively, and the child is dimly recalling the recently renounced experience. Along with the child's present circumstances, these emotional echoes contribute to the shape of the dominant conscious self representation, which is weakened by the reminder of a recently conquered "defect." As the event starts to unfold, this altered self representation remains consciously acceptable, since it is not too discrepant from the original. Still the child has begun to feel tense and somewhat irritable. There is something unpleasant in the air.

What happens next with the young reader depends on how much force the evoked representation has behind it. If his parents drop the suggestion, or if the child loses himself in reading or in some other project, the moment will pass with no dramatic psychological developments. Let us assume, however, that the parents persist and the child is unable to shake off the reverberations of the memory. In these circumstances we can assume that the representation of a younger, weaker self remains dynamically active. The child's feelings turn increasingly unpleasant, and his sense of himself starts to get shaky. The activation of the earlier representation itself has become an emotionally significant event.

Like all events, this one will be subject to representation. The components that will be represented are the dominant conscious self observing (as Freud described in his paper on screen memories) an earlier version of itself in interaction with somebody else. I will call this earlier version *the observed self*. The shapes of the observed self, the object, and the interactional field will not be identical to what they were in the unconscious representation. Like all representations, each is a multiply determined construction. And their shape will be influenced partly by the nature of the original experience but also by current circumstances. This accounts for the tendentiousness of memory that Freud noted and for what I call re-representation.

One implication of this formulation is that there is always a wide range

of possible re-representations of the same evoked memory, depending on current needs, fears, and such, as well as on the qualities of the original experience. The representational world at any moment includes a number of these re-representations, all multiply determined, at varying levels of accessibility to consciousness. It is a function of the ego to compare and to judge the compatibility of various shapes of the self representation. If the shape of the observing self and the shape of the self in the evoked representation are compatible, the subject will have a conscious memory that gives depth and texture to immediate experience. If they are not compatible, conscious awareness of the old image—and of the entire event, including its emotional tone—is impossible. The entire evoked representation is therefore repressed.

For the sake of discussion it is helpful to imagine three versions of the evoked memory. The first is conscious. Following Freud's suggestion that in our conscious memories we stand outside ourselves, we can say that this version contains three components: an observing self, an observed self, and an object. The shape of the observing self has been further modified from what it was when the memory was first evoked, because of the continuing influence of the earlier self representation. It is, however, still close enough to the shape of the dominant self representation to be consciously acceptable. In contrast, the shape of the observed self will have been more powerfully shaped by the evoked experience. The observed self dates from a different time, and its shape was constructed in different circumstances. Let me add quickly that the "different time" needn't have been very long ago. Seeing people several times a week in psychoanalytic treatment gives us an excellent vantage point for observing dramatic shifts in the quality of self representations. These representations often change dramatically from session to session (or even in the course of a single session). The shape of the observed self, despite its difference from the observing self, is also consciously tolerable. Thus this whole version of the experience is present in awareness; it is what Freud would have called a tendentious memory.

Consider the way the child in my example might consciously represent the threatening memory of being read to. He looks upon himself with the sort of disdain that children feel for those they consider babyish. This disdain would be an important element of the shape of the observing self. The child might, if questioned, characterize the experience as "yukky" or "gross." The child in the conscious memory (the observed self) is someone he might once have been, but it certainly has nothing to do with the per-

son he now is. In constructing things like this, he feels strong and in control of himself.

A second version of the evoked memory will be preconscious. Each component of the representation (observing self, observed self, object, and interactional field) has been influenced dramatically by the impact of the old experience. Staying with our example, the new reader's observing self is degraded by the awareness, forced upon it, of its former weakness. The observed self is represented as further deflated, both by the lack of competence (not knowing how to read) and by the passivity (from the perspective of the older child) of his posture toward the parents. The representation of the parents is similarly reshaped in accord with the child's sense of his own degraded participation. They may be experienced as intrusively forcing something on the child, as contemptuous of his incompetence, as enticing the child into a forbidden activity, as begrudging in their involvement, and so on. Finally, the quality of the interactional field itself is deformed—the child doesn't experience himself as participating, but as being imposed upon, regressively indulged, seduced, and so on. The entire representation is colored by an affective tone reflecting the child's sense of shame and humiliation.

The child will defend himself against awareness of this experience in two related ways. First, he will construct a conscious re-representation in which he experiences disdain directed toward anybody (including his earlier self) who would be interested in being read to. In turn, this disdain will be enacted. The child demonstrates his contempt for nonreaders by aggressively refusing to go along with his parents' suggestion that they read aloud. But despite its tenacity, the defense is readily breached; the repression barrier between preconscious and conscious mental contents is permeable.* This theoretical construction reflects observations of the relative ease with which the humiliating experience can be made conscious. Insensitive or harsh parents can mortify their children simply by being persistent. This is also an ever-present danger in clinical work, especially when the analyst is overzealous.

From a dynamic point of view, the preconscious re-representation is both defended against (by the conscious re-representation) and defensive (against more deeply unconscious mental contents). All defense involves

---

*Freud (1900) proposed a "second censorship" between the preconscious and the conscious. Sandler and Sandler (1983, 1987) have developed this concept, both theoretically and clinically, far beyond what Freud had in mind. My formulation has a good deal in common with their three-box model, although there are also considerable differences.

re-representation. This points to a new hypothesis: *Repression begins with and is sustained by the re-representation of evoked events.*

ONE FEATURE of the situation as I have developed it is striking. Conscious and preconscious memories invariably include three representations. There is an observing self (shaped by the child's current needs and attitudes) in addition to the observed self and the object. *Re-represented experience is inevitably triangular.* This accords with Freud's observation that childhood memories include the adult as observer of the child-self. I would carry the idea a step further: what we have seen about the process of re-representation gives us another reason to believe that, when we speak of neurologically intact adults, all conscious and preconscious experience, including the recall of putatively dyadic events, is in fact triangular. The dyad is essentially a fiction—although from the point of view of clinical tactics, it can be useful.

The characteristics of this new triangular experience are the same, in principle, as those of the triangular experiences I discussed in the last chapter. The "person who is not there" in the re-representation is the observed self. The observed self is very different from the person represented as the observing self. Also, because it is a construction drawn from experience distant in time, there is a great deal of fantasy involved in the new representation of the observed self. Consider, for example, a child's perspective on the size of things. We have all had the experience of returning to a long-abandoned childhood place and being amazed by how small everything is. The shock we feel at such moments is a measure of the fundamental discontinuity between what we see now and how things looked when we were small.

To reconnect with our early experience takes considerable empathic (and imaginative) capabilities. It is not overstating the case to say that doing so is tantamount to establishing an object relationship with our child-self. This relationship is significantly colored by our fantasies of who we were then. It is a relationship similar to the one between the observing and the observed self. Needless to say, emotional experience changes as dramatically as physical perspective, and it can do so over much shorter periods of time.

Fantasies about the observed self make it difficult to test early memories against reality, especially when they are emotionally powerful. This is true even if the object of the represented experience is alive, available, and relatively unchanged. That is why patients are often disappointed when they

try to confirm important childhood recollections, even with the coopera-
tion of capable and well-intentioned parents or other relatives.

WE ARE left with those representations that belong to the unconscious
region of the ego. We can think of these as the original representations,
which will be dyadic if they derive from a time before the child became
capable of triangular experience. They can never be experienced directly;
only their derivatives, triangulated and re-represented, can reach consciousness. Accordingly, the observing self does not appear in the unconscious version of the representation. It is added only to preconscious and
conscious re-representations. This is one reason why the repression barrier
between the unconscious and the other regions is far more solid than the
one we have previously encountered. The formulation is in line with
Freud's idea that memories do not emerge but are created.

The shapes of self, object, and interactional field in the unconscious
representation are different from those in the preconscious and conscious
re-representations. In our example they reflect the child's original experience of power, excitement, and exuberance in the act of being read to. At
the moment, the sense of excitement and pleasure are extremely dangerous
to the child, because (subjectively) they seriously threaten the sense of self
built on having achieved a valued capacity. Because the shape of the unconsciously represented self and the shape of the dominant self representation are grossly incompatible, and because the threat of regression is
(again subjectively) very real, there are no available re-representations that
even come close to the excitement and joy the child once felt. Instead,
other conscious and preconscious re-representations defend against awareness of the unconscious version of the event. As a result, the child easily
experiences the shame of being read to (the preconscious re-representation); it is much more difficult for him to become consciously aware of
the exuberance and feelings of power he once felt in that situation.

Although I have focused on the construction of conscious and preconscious re-representations, I do want to mention that new unconscious mental contents are also formed throughout life. This happens when the experience (a wish or an event) contains a self representation grossly
discrepant with the dominant shape of the self. The incompatibility can
be so great that the person is not able to construct a re-representation that
brings the observed and the observing self into the same event. There is
too much fear that the dominant self will be contaminated by the intolerable characteristics of the threatening representation. To the extent that

this situation registers consciously at all, it is probably along the lines of what Sullivan (1953) described as a "not-me" experience. The wish or event is banished to the unconscious without any representation of an observing self. It cannot be experienced directly but will be subject to re-representation in accord with the process I have described.

The Conditions of Re-Representation

The reevaluation of established representations is most likely to occur when a person is in the process of psychological change. So it is most common during childhood, when capacities, interests, attitudes, needs, and passions are most in a state of flux. Freud was working toward the same thought when he came up with the concept of organic repression. Linked to the sequential emergence of leading erogenous zones and modes, the idea of organic repression was that old ways of experiencing pleasure threaten our sense of having matured and grown beyond them.

But organic repression failed theoretically. First, it was overbiologized and too narrowly focused on sexual pleasure as opposed to more broadly based changes in the sense of self. It took no account of change based on the achievement of new capacities, the acquisition of new information through observation of circumstances in general and other people in particular, the formation of new qualities of relatedness, the development of new attitudes, and so on. Second, it was inextricably linked with the notion that there is a developmental end point in adult genitality. This limited Freud's vision both of the sorts of experiences that are likely to be re-represented and of the importance of the process throughout the course of life.*

In contrast, I believe that the sorts of appraisal that lead to re-representation go on constantly. They are particularly apparent at times of emotional upheaval. When people are working hard to make progressive changes in their lives, when they are shaken by loss or intense anxiety, when they are engaged in creative efforts—all of these are occasions for the evocation and re-representation of early experience. The stresses and opportunities of analytic treatment are well suited to destabilize estab-

---

*Freud thought his analogy between memory and a nation's tendentious rewriting applied to childhood memories only. The conscious memories of adulthood, he claimed, tend to be accurate (1910a, p. 84). Observations of patients during the course of analysis make this suggestion questionable at best.

lished representations, a fact that makes analysis particularly useful as an investigative tool.

The oedipal period is a good example of the kind of upheaval that leads to broadly based re-representation and to the repression of a great deal of what went before. Consider the seductive sexual approaches that oedipal children make toward their parents. I don't agree with the received psychoanalytic wisdom that these advances begin at age three or four; certainly they start much earlier. But we do know that something changes at three or four: by then the child is old enough to conceptualize and represent triangular relationships. Previously, so long as the child's experience of his approach involved only two people (the child and the object of his advances), the experience could be enjoyed unambivalently. As his cognitive and imaginative capacities develop, however, he becomes aware of the reactions of the other parent to what is going on.

This new awareness colors the child's feelings about the sexual approaches. Just what he will feel about them is variable, depending largely on his experience of the absent parent. If the father is seen as destructible, the child will feel triumphant or guilty; if the child believes him to be punitive, he will feel anxious or ashamed; if the parent is seen as too encouraging, the child will feel that his autonomy has been usurped. Whatever the particulars, seduction can never be the same once experience has been triangulated.

The representational model makes it clear that past exchanges will be reevaluated in terms of later knowledge. It is not, "That was all right then, but it's not all right now." Rather, everything in the child's conscious and preconscious experience is recast so that it was never all right in the first place. This tendentious revision of earlier experience happens whenever early representations are repressed and re-representations are constructed.

The example of the oedipal child emphasizes changes that derive from maturational advances in the child's cognitive capacities. These advances make triangulation possible and decisively recast the early experiences. Other internal changes bring about the same results, especially ebbs and flows in the force of motives organized around the workings of the safety and effectance drives. It is reasonable to assume that the relative strength of safety and effectance needs is in a state of flux throughout the course of life. As the balance shifts, and as old aims are abandoned and new ones emerge, early experience is constantly reassessed.

It is not only changing abilities and developmental needs that instigate re-representation. It can also be the result of what the child learns over

time about his objects. He may learn something new because he has become a more sophisticated observer—he notices something that was there all along but that he was too young to notice before. Or the parent's reaction itself may change over time. Some parents are able to enjoy and encourage the child's ambitions and his achievement of new capabilities when the child is very young. The child will represent events organized around his effectance strivings very positively for a time—they bring him and his parents together, leading to highly valued self representations and to affectionate representations of the object. But as the child develops and his ambitions become more of a direct challenge, the parents may become more threatened. Perhaps they feel that their own sense of competence is endangered by the child's developing abilities and his ambitions to use them, or they feel the stirrings of separation anxiety when they sense that the child will one day leave. Not infrequently it happens that the child will capitalize on his new strength to express old hostile feelings toward the parents, a change that the parents register, at least preconsciously.

In each of these circumstances, the child will come to feel increasingly guilty and anxious about expressing his ambition. This leads not only to more ambivalent reactions to present events, but also to reappraisal of the evoked representations of events organized around the early ambitious strivings. The child will of course recall examples of interpersonal situations that explain the feelings. At the same time, he will lose the idea that what is now shrouded in anxiety and guilt was once exciting and pleasurable. Later it will be a goal of his analysis to work through the various re-representations that color his weakened, guilty sense of himself, and to get closer to those that more closely approximate the original sense of himself as enjoying his ambitions and achievements.*

The Representational Model and Clinical Process

In this chapter and the last I have constructed a model that reflects my way of working as a psychoanalyst. I believe that the model also offers a useful way of thinking about what happens in treatment to facilitate

---

*This line of thought illuminates what I consider an important shortcoming in Kohut's psychology of the self. Kohut assumed that an inhibition of ambition results from the parents' early failure to mirror the child's grandiosity. In contrast I believe that the inhibition may emerge later in life and only retroactively color earlier experience. Also, any memories of failed mirroring are themselves re-representations that must be understood on the basis of subsequent dynamic developments.

change. In the next chapters I will develop some of the technical implications of this perspective. For the moment, let me make a brief comment
on the relation between my theoretical structure and the therapeutic goals
of analytic treatment.

I agree, broadly, with Freud that analyzable psychopathology is the result of the repression of emotionally powerful mental contents. Experience
is constricted and deformed when we cannot become aware of the wide
range of motives that move us or of the representations that guide us. We
act most freely, creatively, and effectively when we have access to as much
as possible of our inner lives. Without that access our sense of ourselves
and others is compromised, and our actions are likely to be self-defeating.

A central premise of the model I have proposed is that any emotionally
significant event will generate, at different times and in different circumstances, many re-representations. The range of re-representations reaching
consciousness at any time depends on the shape and flexibility of the dominant self representation. Benign changes in either shape or flexibility
make it possible for people to accept an increasing variety of previously
intolerable re-representations. As self experience becomes less rigid, more
evoked representations will be acceptable.

This formulation suggests to me that the analytic process follows two
tracks, conceptually independent but pragmatically inseparable. First,
work is directed at increasing the flexibility of the dominant self representations. The work involves facilitating the patient's sense of safety in the
face of emerging transference experiences that evoke dangerous archaic
experiences and intolerable re-representations. When this aspect of the
work has gone well, the patient is able to maintain his self-assurance while
confronting an increasing variety of self representations. He is able to tolerate the idea that he can be sexual or ambitious or dependent or murder-
ously angry—all possibilities previously disowned. The range of what he
allows himself to think (about himself and others) expands greatly as the
result of this element of analytic treatment.

Changes in the flexibility of the dominant self representation occur
largely in response to the personal influence of the analyst. Whether we
refer to the holding function of the analyst (Winnicott, 1963), the analytic
frame (Khan, 1960), the analyst's role as an auxiliary superego (Strachey,
1934), or the analytic attitude (Schafer, 1983), the unique nature of the
analyst's presence has long been seen as the crucial force in facilitating a
patient's ability to risk expanded awareness of previously rejected mental
contents. The representational model suggests that the analyst's influence

is most effective in increasing the patient's sense of safety, thereby facilitating greater flexibility in the dominant self representation.

At the same time, the representational model makes it clear that there are limits to how influential the analyst's personal presence can be. Especially in recent years, there has been an assumption that patients will respond quickly and easily to particular behaviors of the analyst and that this can be substantially therapeutic in its own right. Thus Kohut (1971, 1984) argues for the therapeutic power of the analyst's empathy, and Weiss, Sampson, and their colleagues (1986) believe that the analyst's actions can disconfirm the "pathogenic beliefs" at the core of neurosis.

In contrast, my conviction that all re-representation—all experience that can become preconscious or conscious—is triangular makes it difficult to attribute so much power to the analyst. According to some theorists, if the analyst reacts enthusiastically or affirmatively (or neutrally, for that matter) to the patient's pursuit of chronically conflicted goals, she will offer the patient an alternative to the experience that has been stored as a representation and that tends to be evoked whenever the patient is moved to pursue those goals. In response, the patient will have a new store of experience to draw upon that will correct the old assumptions.

If representations were dyadic, the new relationship with the analyst might correct previous expectations. But recall the characteristics of triangular experience: there is always a powerful but elusive relationship with the absent third person. In the case of re-representations, the "absent third person" is the observed self, and that representation is highly colored by fantasy, making the re-represented experience resistant to correction or even to reality testing.

Consider the patient struggling with her ambitious strivings described earlier. The observed self in re-representations of times when she felt or acted ambitiously was represented as messy and destructive. The analyst's attitude toward the patient's ambitions *in the present* cannot affect the shape of the observed self, which was formed by past experience and is now strongly influenced by fantasy. And since the shape of the observed self is an important determinant of the shape of the observing self, the analyst's power to change even that must remain limited. Thus the patient's self-experience has a momentum behind it that resists rectification by subsequent experience. What the analyst can do is to address the dominant sense of self in a way that makes it increasingly safe to experience the previously rejected re-representations.

This leads to the second aspect of the analytic process. The analyst facilitates the patient's ability to grasp the content of representations that were previously warded off by defensively constructed re-representations. This is more familiar as the interpretive process itself; the analyst risks her own guesses about the content of rejected representations. This has two results. First, the patient is able to get progressively closer to the original repressed representations (although never to any direct recall of them). Second, perhaps more important, he is able to become aware of more and more of the previously rejected re-representations that color everyday experience. He learns more about the depth and richness of his life.

Remaining with the patient struggling with ambition, we begin by acknowledging the conscious re-representations that ward off preconscious representations of the self as destructive, aggressive, perversely sexual, or messy in a variety of other ways. From there, we interpret the preconscious re-representations, which include the observing self reshaped by its humiliating and anxiety-ridden awareness of the forbidden characteristics. Finally, we get closer to the more deeply unconscious versions of the representation, arriving eventually at the self excited and expansive about expressions of ambition. Through working on these various re-representations, patient and analyst come to understand the dynamic relationships among them—especially the way that each re-representation can function as a defense, limiting awareness of other perspectives on the patient's experience. Ultimately they will also come to a deeper appreciation of the patient's motivational conflicts. They will see the clash between safety and effectance motives and the role these have come to play in the formation of the representations themselves.

Throughout this discussion I have focused on the increasing awareness of a range of representations of the self. This reflects the idea that guarding the sense of self is the fundamental motive for repression. It should be clear that the work of interpretation is also directed at warded-off representations of the object. Awareness of forbidden impressions of the object can be a source of anxiety or guilt in its own right, either because something forbidden has been observed or because the act of observation itself is off limits. This aspect of the neurotic process and its analysis is complementary to what I have already described. In Chapter 10 I will return to the problem and develop it in my discussions of transference and countertransference.

Because emotionally powerful events generate so many re-representa-

tions, it makes no sense to say that analysis ever reaches an end point. It is more accurate to see the process as one of cycling through a shifting field of linked experiences, never passing from distortion to historical truth, but always working toward a deeper understanding of the patient's unique way of making sense of and coping with experience. This reflects what it feels like to do an analysis, and I believe it is a process well captured by my representational model.

Technical Implications

Theoretical Models and the Analyst's Neutrality

SINCE Breuer first met Anna O., psychoanalysts have struggled to understand the relationship between analyst and analysand. The attempt has been both urgent and elusive. It is urgent not only because clinicians need practical guidelines but also because a relationship so powerful cries out for some rationale. Without one, visions of alchemy loom large. It is elusive because, like all lengthy, intimate interpersonal involvements, it defies simple description, much less full comprehension. Freud could be uncharacteristically diffident when he talked about how the analyst's presence influenced the treatment process. His comparison of technique to the rules of chess, emphasizing the infinite variability of procedures during the prolonged middle phase of analysis, suggests that full systematization is impossible and probably not even desirable.

In Chapter 8 I sketched out a two-track formulation of the psychoanalytic process. First, the analyst works to facilitate the feeling of safety that allows the observing self to tolerate more and more of the re-representations of early experience that had been warded off. When this happens, the dominant self representation becomes increasingly flexible, and the patient can risk awareness of previously intolerable ways of thinking. Only in the context of the feeling of safety can patient and analyst follow the second track, putting words to the re-representations that emerge. This process requires interpretation of the patient's experience, especially within the transference, and constitutes what has traditionally been seen as the core of psychoanalytic treatment.

In this chapter I will discuss some ideas about how the analysis can promote therapeutic change in the observing self. This depends to a great extent on the quality of the relationship between analyst and analysand, so

I will address the implications of my representational model for the analyst's stance. I will be particularly concerned with the much maligned but, as I hope to demonstrate, still useful concept of analytic neutrality.

Neutrality in the Drive Model

Freud's vision of the analyst's stance is based on the position of the observing scientist as it was understood in the nineteenth century. The Spanish philosopher Ortega y Gasset characterized this scientific attitude:

> At last man is to know the truth about everything. It suffices that he should not lose heart at the complexity of the problems, and that he should allow no passion to cloud his mind. If with serene self-mastery he uses the apparatus of his intellect, if in particular he uses it in orderly fashion, he will find that his faculty of thought is *ratio,* reason, and that in reason he possesses the almost magic power of reducing everything to clarity, of turning what is most opaque to crystal, penetrating it by analysis until it is become self-evident (1941, pp. 170–171).

Freud aspired to just the sort of dispassionate clarity that Ortega mocked. Science, he believed, can rise above all other mental activities, laying a unique claim to objectivity. In a letter to Theodore Reik he wrote: "scientific research . . . must be without presumptions. In every other kind of thinking the choice of a point of view cannot be avoided" (1928, p. 196).

The comment embodies a notion about science that contemporary philosophers (and scientists as well) consider outmoded and even presumptuous. Derived from the Cartesian belief in the separability of observer and observed, it envisions the possibility of data uncontaminated by presumption and of theories derived from the data by the application of unbiased rationality. Scientists stand apart from their subject, viewing the phenomena with a special kind of detachment. It is this very detachment that allows the impartial application of reason and facilitates the emergence of truth.

Freud's commitment to the idealized nineteenth-century vision of science was deeply felt, but it also had its political side. Throughout his life an important aim of his writing was to establish the legitimacy of psychoanalysis, both as an intellectual discipline and as a treatment method. From the beginning, both goals were challenged by charges that the entire process was contaminated by suggestion: the analyst was simply planting ideas in his patient's head. Thus the data of psychoanalysis were worthless,

the apparent effects of treatment could be explained as the results of coercion, and the entire undertaking was conceptually (perhaps even morally) tainted.

Many of Freud's technical prescriptions address this concern, at least implicitly. Read in context they turn out to be responses to the idea that suggestion by the analyst is responsible both for therapeutic change and for the data on which analytic theory is based. The posture of "evenly hovering attention," the "blank screen" or "reflecting mirror" analogies, and the suggestion of an attitude of "surgical detachment" (Freud, 1913) all reflect Freud's contention that the analyst can be no different from any other scientist of the day.

The neutral analyst as Freud envisioned him is an outsider impartially observing his patient's passions, prohibitions, fears, and compromises. Freud himself used the term "neutrality" rarely and narrowly. It first appears in the context of advice to analysts about how to handle patients' declarations of love. Responding in kind, whether encouragingly or discouragingly, will defeat the analysis, Freud warns, and he goes on to say that "we ought not to give up the neutrality toward the patient, which we have acquired through keeping the counter-transference in check" (1915d, p. 164). Freud went no further in spelling out what he intended neutrality to mean. In fact, despite being a keystone of the traditional conceptualization of the analytic posture, a formal definition of neutrality did not appear until Anna Freud suggested one in 1936. In *The Ego and the Mechanisms of Defense* she wrote:

> It is the task of the analyst to bring into consciousness that which is unconscious, no matter to which psychic institution it belongs. He directs his attention equally and objectively to the unconscious elements in all three institutions. To put it in another way, when he sets about the work of enlightenment, he takes his stand at a point equidistant from the id, the ego, and the superego (1936, p. 28).

Notice in this the assumptions of objectivity borne of externality, the rationality leading to enlightenment, the impartiality of the reasonable observer. Poland gives externality a clinical slant: "Neutrality is the technical manifestation of respect for the essential otherness of the patient" (1984, p. 289).

Although Anna Freud's definition sounds precise enough, it resists transformation into behavioral terms. How does the neutral analyst *act*? Among those currently relying on neutrality as the keystone of a correct

clinical posture, there remains confusion about how it is best expressed within the psychoanalytic situation. There is general agreement that the analyst should try not to impose his values on the patient and that he should keep his countertransference in check. The plot thickens, however, when it comes to realizing these attitudes in terms of technical procedures. Myerson (1981b) goes so far as to acknowledge that neutrality is virtually impossible to define in behavioral terms. Observing a session, we would find little consensus about whether an analyst is being neutral; it is difficult to relate neutrality to factors such as the analyst's level of responsiveness, expressions of encouragement, or enforcement of conditions of abstinence (see Panel, 1984).

Yet there is a broad tendency among authors who use the term to translate neutrality into behaviors such as nonresponsiveness or anonymity. To understand why, consider what we find in the *Oxford English Dictionary*. For the analyst, the first definition of *neutral* is both useful and dangerous: "Not assisting, or actively taking the side of, either party in the case of a war or disagreement between other states; remaining inactive in relation to the belligerent powers." This is close to what Anna Freud had in mind, but note the stress on inactivity. This has led to difficulties with the term, even among those who endorse its goals.

Some analysts believe that impartiality is best achieved through inactivity. But what does it mean to be inactive in a relationship? Subsequent definitions in the dictionary add connotations of indifference and colorlessness. Are these the route to inactivity? If they are, then as a summary statement of an analytic stance "neutrality" is a weak, bloodless term. It fails to capture the emotional intensity of the clinical encounter. Many analysts feel that the term is too cold, that it does not convey the kind of affirmation or engagement that patients typically get in a well-conducted treatment.

Why should psychoanalysis be stuck with a concept that ties impartial acceptance of all parts of the patient's personality to the analyst's inactivity and nonexpressiveness? The reason, I believe, is traceable to neutrality's roots in the epistemological premises of the drive model. There is a direct line from the Cartesian stress on the observer's objectivity to the drive model's equation of nonalignment to nonparticipation. Inactivity in the interest of discovery is at least an apparently logical next step.

These difficulties with prescriptive definitions lead me to suggest that neutrality should not be thought of as a behavioral concept at all. Interpreting, remaining silent, maintaining anonymity, or giving advice refer

to possible behaviors of the analyst. Neutrality, on the other hand, is most useful as a way of talking about a particular therapeutic *form*—or, to put it differently, it is a way of understanding the *goal* of the analyst's behavior. It is a word like "democracy," which refers to a kind of government rather than to the particular laws that implement it. Once we have consensus about what a word like democracy means, we can debate how desirable it is compared with other kinds of government. The status of the neutrality concept should be similar. When we have achieved some sort of agreement about what neutrality is, we will be free to discuss when and whether it is an appropriate goal, and consensus as to its desirability still leaves open the question of how to achieve it.

The Relational Critique of Neutrality

Even if we accept the idea that neutrality should refer to a goal rather than to a behavior, there are problems with the concept. Despite its connections with objectivity and rationality, "neutrality" itself is far from a neutral word: any definition inevitably changes with alterations in the underlying theory. When Freud first introduced the term, he was talking about the need for the analyst to resist countertransferential pressures. He was not talking about equidistance from psychological structures, as Anna Freud was in her definition, nor could he have constructed the concept in those terms. At the time of the technical papers, Freud was working with the topographic model; the mind was divided into the systems Ucs., Pcs., and Cs. The analyst in this model was explicitly allied with the Ucs.; the very goal of analysis was to make the unconscious conscious. Any notion of equidistance awaited a crucial theoretical change: the tripartite structural model with its idea that there are unconscious elements in all psychic structures.

In fact, Anna Freud's formulation is not simply a plea for fair-mindedness. The classic definition appears in the context of her argument for the legitimacy of studying and analyzing the ego. Her polemic was directed against the large number of analysts who refused to abandon the older system, in which ego functioning was considered the sort of superficial study that could be of interest only to academic psychologists (Lichtenberg, 1983b).

The analyst's neutrality can be evaluated only from within a particular theoretical system. Accordingly, the most telling critique of the concept has come from analysts working within the relational model. Based not

on Cartesian rationalism but on a philosophy of science informed by Heisenberg's uncertainty principle and Einstein's relativity theory, the relational model postulates an analyst who is, in Sullivan's phrase, a "participant observer" or, in Fairbairn's, an "interventionist." These concepts are not themselves technical prescriptions (suggestions that one *ought* to participate or to intervene); they are statements of fact from a particular philosophical perspective. Theorists who disagree on many other issues unite in insisting that the analyst inevitably participates, inevitably reveals himself, inevitably influences the course of treatment and the evolution of the transference. This perspective is forcefully stated by Wachtel: "So-called neutrality is but one more way of participating in the events of the therapeutic process, and is no less likely to influence ensuing events than any other way of participating" (1982, p. 263).

Arguments stressing the inevitability of the analyst's participation—what Hoffman (1983) and Gill (1983b) have called the radical critique of the blank-screen position—rest on very strong grounds. There are two people in the room during every analytic session. Storytellers, historians, and even contemporary physicists are fully aware that no data-gathering enterprise is free from the influence of the data gatherer. Spence (1982) and Schafer (1980, 1983) have advanced particularly compelling accounts of the effects that the analyst's preferred narrative structure has on the course of treatment. But the relational critique opens a Pandora's box. Wachtel argues that, since neutrality is simply one way among many of participating in the therapeutic interaction, it has no special claim to legitimacy. Active (behavioral) techniques, which are themselves simply therapeutically effective ways of participating, are no less neutral than neutrality. It is then only a small step from the idea of influence to active approaches that endorse the analyst's using his influence to bring about particular therapeutic goals. While Wachtel is principally concerned with symptomatic improvement, more subtle interventions are tempting. Analysts who remain committed to an exploratory approach may use their influence to help the patient to tolerate intimacy or to express feelings more freely or to individuate with less conflict.

This use of the analyst's participation amounts to therapeutic zeal and is incompatible with the analytic goals I described in Chapter 8. It is detrimental to the goal of self-knowledge because it encourages the dissociation of crucial aspects of the patient's personality—aspects that may be regressive, masochistic, destructive, or rebellious. If the analyst clearly values a particular sort of change, the patient can come to feel that acceptance

by the analyst is contingent upon the patient's being collaborative and making progress. The analyst can inadvertently become a kind of critical observing self, creating an atmosphere in which important aspects of the transference may be irretrievably lost. In contrast, the atmosphere embodied in the concept of neutrality is one in which the analyst is distinctly on the side of the patient, but not on the side of one aspect of the patient's personality at the expense of others. There is no pretense that the patient's associations can unfold as if she were the only person in the consulting room but, realizing this, the analyst can attempt to be a benign and affirmative presence. The analyst's influence is inevitable, but it should be directed toward helping the patient to acknowledge the various aspects of her personality—her impulses as much as her defenses, her kindness as much as her vindictiveness, her hated as much as her loved self and object representations, her regressive as well as her progressive tendencies. Only within this kind of atmosphere can the patient gain the freedom to know herself.

The relational critique highlights a serious dilemma inherent in conceptualizing the analyst's stance. Neutrality as developed within the drive model embodies respect for the patient's autonomy and freedom to express all sides of the personality without concern for the analyst's preferences. But it is weak at conceptualizing the analyst's personal influence on the treatment process. In sharp contrast, the relational vision of the analyst as inevitable participant sensitizes us to his influence but makes it difficult to justify his impartiality, especially in the face of the patient's pathological or regressive tendencies.

A Representational Approach to Neutrality

The representational model I have developed suggests both the inevitability of the analyst's participation in the clinical process and the therapeutic value of his impartiality. The model lends itself to a structural vision of a neutral analytic stance in Anna Freud's sense of equidistance. However, since it is based on radically different epistemological and psychodynamic principles than the drive model, the representational model requires a new definition of the term. Epistemologically, the model is not built on Freud's rationalism. The key to this is in the way I have used the concept "representation" itself; it is defined as a multiply determined construction influenced by inner needs and by interpersonal perception. Thus the model holds that the nuances of the analyst's participation will be apparent to the

patient and will significantly shape the entire analytic experience. Similarly, the analyst's experience of the patient will be shaped by his own internal processes (prior experience, needs, theoretical commitments, and so on). The analyst has neither a bias-free theory nor a capacity for pristine empathy that gives him any unmediated access to the "truth" about the patient.

Dynamically, the representational model does not see the analyst struggling to maintain impartiality among the surging passions of the id, the stern prohibitions of the superego, and the adaptive or defensive compromises of the ego. The contents of the mind are the various sorts of representations that encode our experience: the dominant self representation; wishes shaped by the safety and effectance drives; the evoked representations of self and object in relation with each other; and the multilayered re-representations they generate. When conflicts develop, they involve those representations that are tolerable to the dominant self representation, and therefore capable of becoming conscious, and those that are not. The analyst participating with the patient creates events that constantly and inevitably evoke a range of re-representations. Some of these support the dominant sense of self and are experienced as safe. Others threaten the sense of self and are experienced as dangerous.

When the analyst is experienced as safe, his presence promotes a sense of well-being that influences the shape of the dominant self representation. This creates the analytic atmosphere that makes treatment possible. Only under conditions of perceived security can the patient risk elaborating the thoughts, fantasies, and feelings that need to be brought to light and examined if analysis is to proceed beneficially (see Myerson, 1981a, 1981b). Without feeling safe the patient could not, as Schafer puts it, "take on what he or she ventures to confront during the analysis, and instead would continue simply to feel injured, betrayed, threatened, seduced, or otherwise interfered with or traumatized" (1983, p. 32).

Notice that Schafer says that the patient would *continue* to feel injured and so on. He is referring to the potential, in every analysis, for the patient to believe that the analyst is similar or even identical to the dangerous objects of her early experience. The representational model suggests that this will happen when there is something in the analytic relationship that is reminiscent of the archaic experiences. The evoked events further color the patient's transference experience, so that the analyst becomes indistinguishable from the original dangerous objects. The patient is left where she started, trapped in yet another hopeless situation. To avoid this, the

analyst must *do something* to differentiate himself from the old object. It is in this doing that neutrality is established. In agreement with Schafer, then, I see a close connection between the analyst's neutrality and the patient's experience of safety.

Ironically, however, the analyst cannot be experienced as too safe or as too allied with the dominant self representation. He must be wary not simply to gratify the patient's safety needs, since then the patient's experience in the analysis will not be similar enough to old repressed events to evoke a wide range of re-representations. There will be no room for transference, with all the dangers entailed by the eruption of threatening feelings within the context of an archaic relationship. Many patients—and, I hasten to add, some analysts too—eagerly and defensively embrace the analyst's tendency to position himself as a safe object. They embrace the tendency eagerly because there is genuine relief from a life of relationships gone awry; they embrace him defensively because the "good" therapeutic relationship temporarily defuses conflict. But the analyst who is too much a safe object has fallen into a trap; he inhibits the evocation of those re-representations that give shape to the patient's transference, especially the negative transference.

I am suggesting here that there is a need to strike a kind of balance between the patient's experience of the analyst as a safe and as a dangerous presence. This recalls Anna Freud's idea of neutrality as equidistance, although when addressing operations within the representational world I prefer a term like "optimal tension" because of its dynamic connotations. With this in mind, I think we can define neutrality from the perspective of the representational model: *The neutral analyst occupies a position that maintains an optimal tension between the patient's tendency to see him as a dangerous object and the capacity to experience him as a safe one.*

The importance of achieving a neutral stance is closely related to Schafer's beautifully stated formulation of ego syntonicity:

> the concept of ego-syntonicity has always referred to those principles of constructing experience which seem to be beyond effective question by the person who develops and applies them . . . Metaphorically, they are the eye that sees everything according to its structure and cannot see itself seeing . . . One might say that these principles are beyond question in so far as the person treats the relevant questions about them *not as questions but as evidence* . . . In undertaking the analysis of a character problem, one counts on there being some diversity of experiential principles . . . The point of access may be some well-guarded form of thinking hopefully, some shrugged-off way of esteem-

ing oneself realistically, or some shyly hidden but stable kind of loving (1983, pp. 144–146).

Schafer's point applies equally to the representational world of many patients. The patient can become aware that he is assimilating the analyst into his world of archaic internal objects only when he has already become aware that there is an alternative possibility. Unless he has some sense of the analyst as a safe object, he will not be able to experience him as a dangerous one. The inability to achieve this balance is responsible for many analytic failures. If the analyst cannot be experienced as a safe object, analysis never gets under way; if he cannot be experienced as a dangerous one, it never ends.

Neutrality and Technical Procedure

This revised definition of neutrality has important technical implications. Perhaps most important, we can no longer assume that the same behaviors will implement the goal of neutrality with all patients. This contrasts sharply with the premises of the drive model. In that model, neutrality has a static ring to it because the forces competing for expression are presumed universal. From one analysis to another, the neutral posture would always look more or less the same, at least in our work with "analyzable" patients. This accords well with the model of analyst as nineteenth-century scientist.

But all this changes when we think in terms of representations and re-representations—the old and new, or dangerous and safe, experiences that make up the mental contents of particular individuals. The analyst must tailor his posture to fit the particular representational world that is the unique personal construction of each patient. Accordingly, the behaviors that implement the goal of neutrality are never the same for any two patients. We modify what we do to meet the needs of particular people, and we judge the effectiveness of our interventions by whether they facilitate or inhibit the patient's capacity to risk awareness of new representations.

Under my proposed reformulation, the most important determinant of the activity of the neutral analyst will be the quality of the patient's relationships with others. The analytic behaviors that implement the goal of optimal tension between old and new necessarily vary with the openness to new experience of a particular patient's internal object world. Generally speaking, the silence and anonymity of unmodified classical technique en-

able the patient to include the analyst in her internal object world, while a more active or self-revealing posture establish the analyst as a new object. Thus, with a patient who is firmly encased in a closed world of internal objects, the analyst will have to assert his newness more affirmatively to achieve an optimal level of tension, while with the more open patient just such assertiveness would constitute an impediment to the development of transference and to insight about it. Neutrality is thus not to be measured by the analyst's behavior at any moment, but by the particular patient's ability both to become aware of and to tolerate the transference, as well as other aspects of her experience.

I believe that these considerations cast analytic behaviors such as emotional openness, self-revelation, and even expressing judgments in a new light. These behaviors, which are typically thought of as prima facie non-neutral, may actually contribute to neutrality when judiciously applied with the right patient. Conversely, the strictly interpretive posture that for many analysts defines neutrality may work against it with some patients.

Rather than insisting on a uniform vision of the analyst stance—a notion more honored in the breach anyway—we can tailor it to what we learn about its effects on each patient's self-experience. There are many patients for whom analytic reserve is simply too close to the aloof, self-protective posture with which their parents guarded themselves against their children's erotic, competitive, challenging, or hostile impulses. Then reserve and anonymity can actually detract from neutrality, by confirming the patient's sense of having harmed the analyst. For all intents and purposes, the patient's rage turns the analyst into the damaged, archaic object. Self-revelation can be the road back to neutrality in these circumstances. This is an especially likely situation in the case of the patient who is most locked into the constraints of her internal object world.

Along the same lines, there are some patients who were exposed to parental indifference bordering on neglect. Then the traditionally neutral nonjudgmental attitude can be genuinely dangerous. In these circumstances, passing judgment on the patient's behavior (calling it provocative or self-destructive) or on important people in the patient's life (a disturbed or cruel lover or relative) can be essential to the establishment of neutrality. Schafer is referring to something similar when he says, "It is not a departure from neutrality to call a spade a spade" (1983, p. 6).

Other situations depend less on the patient's representational world and more on the events of the analysis itself. At times, personal revelation may contribute to the establishment, consolidation, or restoration of the neu-

tral atmosphere. There are situations even in otherwise smoothly running analyses when the analyst's countertransference temporarily dominates work on a particular issue. The analyst may have become particularly involved in the patient's ruminations over aspects of his life: should he take the job, marry the woman, continue in treatment. The analyst has come to a clear, although not necessarily objective, point of view on the issue but in the interest of anonymity is withholding it. What develops is a kind of analytic nagging—when the patient expresses feelings different from the analyst's own, the analyst questions relentlessly but hears nothing. The patient digs in, feels a certain amount of despair, and disqualifies an otherwise respected analyst from being of any particular help. Now it can be useful for the analyst to reveal something about himself, his feelings on the issue and perhaps whatever he can figure out about the reasons for those feelings and why they have led to a passive confrontation with the patient. This kind of revelation, which often leads to the discovery of disclaimed aspects of the patient's own feelings, can get the treatment back on an even—from my perspective, neutral—keel.

What I am saying is not startling from the perspective of what analysts actually do. Nothing that we know of what Freud did with his patients suggests that he was anything other than a vibrant and forceful presence in the room. More recently, Ralph Greenson's (1967) concept of the working alliance has pointed to behaviors that encourage a positive relationship between patient and analyst. But this working alliance is explicitly construed as a departure from neutrality, since it represents a collaboration with one part of the patient's psychic structure, the observing ego, at the expense of the other systems. Freud himself made no effort to integrate his frequent personal revelations into his theory of technique. My view of neutrality, however, does make it possible to encompass what Freud, Greenson and many other analysts actually do into a framework that maintains the unique benefits of psychoanalysis as a therapeutic modality.

Let me add a brief warning about the dangers of personal revelation. These are apparent to many analysts and have been frequently discussed in the literature. Poland has well expressed some of the pitfalls, pointing out that analysts often avoid the brunt of their patients' transferential rage by hastening to repair a presumed disappointment. Personal revelations may serve this reparative function, but they often detract from the goal of neutrality. Poland suggests: "Too often this supposedly humane response is a failure of empathic perceptive accuracy. An atmosphere of acceptance

implies full openness; it does not provide a selective filter for the comfort of the analyst" (1984, p. 290).

A related point deserves mention. Frequently, when personal information is given to the patient, unless it comes from a countertransferential outburst, it is given in the interest of promoting either trust or some kind of identification. These goals are generally incompatible with the establishment of a neutral atmosphere because they embody the analyst's decision that he should support or bolster one aspect of the patient's tendencies at the expense of another. Unsurprisingly, the effect of many personal revelations is to stifle feelings. The analyst who has told his patient that he, like the patient, becomes anxious when doing creative work such as writing may intend to promote, through identification, the patient's tolerance for his own anxiety in similar situations—but he will run the risk of making it difficult for the patient to express contempt for the analyst's nonproductivity. The analyst who has told the patient that he has children to whom he is devoted may well have deprived the patient of the freedom to express her hatred for the children who, until that moment, had existed for her only in fantasy. The way I have reformulated neutrality shifts attention from preformed rules of technique to individual clinical judgment. The value of a particular intervention cannot be judged by a theoretical standard, but by whether it promotes risk taking or stultifies the patient. This clinical method is similar to the research protocol employed by Weiss, Sampson, and their colleagues (1986). In their work, they judge the effectiveness of analytic interventions by observing the patient's capacity to introduce new themes. If the patient is able to elaborate ideas about himself or others that he hadn't been able to address before, the intervention has been useful. If not, it has been a failure.

I WILL conclude with an example of the sort of behavior that can support neutrality within the terms of my representational model. The patient is a middle-aged married man who came to analysis because of an obsession about a woman with whom he had recently had a brief flirtation that came to nothing. Although he presented himself as simply wanting to be rid of thoughts about the woman, with very little encouragement he started to care less about the obsession itself and to become more interested in a sense of chronic dissatisfaction with his life both at home and at work.

Within a relatively short time, some fairly dramatic improvements occurred in this man's life. The obsession disappeared, but more important

he began to feel generally open to people in a way that he described as making life far richer than it had been. The scope of his involvement with people and activities grew dramatically. He reported liking himself better and being less anxiously self-absorbed. He acquired new interests.

Despite all these changes, the patient felt that there was a distance between him and me that placed limits on full self-exploration and his growth within the analysis. He felt that he had no relationship with me, that I was distant, aloof, and inscrutable. I didn't answer his questions, preferring instead to demand (as he saw it) his fantasies. Also he objected to my way of running my practice. He could not see why I charged for missed sessions. He could understand being charged if he missed for frivolous reasons, but when he did miss it was always unavoidable. And why didn't I even tell him *why* I did what I did, beyond brief references to my need for some financial stability? Was I just a small-minded cheapskate who hid behind the convenient mask of analytic anonymity?

As the work proceeded, more details of the transference emerged. My failure to answer questions and the demand for fantasies was fundamentally a sadistic and voyeuristic exercise for me: I loved to see him squirm and to come up with fantasies that were wrong. Also I used both my sadism and my analytic status to protect myself from his own assaults—fundamentally, I was afraid of him and, more pointedly, afraid of my own weakness.

The elaboration of these fantasies was essentially affectless. The patient could not allow himself to feel very much about what was emerging because he was convinced that what he saw was true. We were able to connect the fantasies historically to his perception of his father, a weak, frightened man who had been jilted by his mother and who had carried a torch for her all his life. The father had taken a great deal of his helpless anger out on his son—from criticizing the size of his penis and taking him for hormone shots as a small child to denigrating his very real school and work accomplishments later on. Still there was no real involvement. We both learned a good deal as we constructed his transferential feelings in terms of defense against and recreation of his relationship with his father, but nothing much changed. The bottom line for the patient was that I *was* like his father or, as he put it other times, *analysis* was too much like his father.

Over time I came to believe that perhaps these complaints were justified; perhaps unmodified anonymity *was* too much like the begrudging, self-protective attitude the patient had experienced as coming from his

father. This led to a change in tone in the sessions. During one exchange about some sessions canceled because of bad weather, the patient again asked me why I persisted in the small-minded practice of charging him when I knew perfectly well that he had a good reason for not coming. This time I told him that, although I had no doubt that it would have been extremely difficult for him to make the appointments, I charged him because I didn't want to be in the position of judging whether he had good reasons or not. Further I said that it would be disrespectful for me to judge the validity of his reasons for missing a session on any particular occasion and I felt most comfortable simply relying on guidelines established in advance.

The patient, surprised and pleased, responded, "Oh, why didn't you tell me that before?" I said it was because I hadn't thought it would be helpful, but perhaps I was wrong. This opened up a period of sustained anger—the first expressions of anger beyond the potshots or hit-and-run attacks that characterized the earlier work.

During this period, which lasted for several weeks, the patient thought seriously of ending the analysis. Why had I been so like his father for so long, and why should he have to put up with and suffer for my mistakes? He also was clearly afraid of what he was feeling. He speculated that maybe it was all for the good, that it was better to feel something for me than nothing. He sought reassurance that this was a sign of analytic progress, but I wasn't entirely sure myself that it was. In fact, I said, it was possible that the anger was a first step in ending the analysis, that it was something to be taken very seriously.

But the anger subsided, and the patient was able to react more directly to my having told him why I charged for the session and, more important, that I respected him. His reaction was of course not unambivalent. He had a dream in which he, an avid tennis player, was playing with John McEnroe. He had the sense that he could beat McEnroe, or at least give him a good game, but he noticed that although several of his shots were out McEnroe was calling them good. He was able to hear and elaborate my interpretation—that he felt I was toying with him, letting him think he was in my league, building him up for a harsh disappointment. This was the first time that he was able to connect in a full emotional way with a transferential implication of one of his dreams.

In the context of these exchanges, the patient rather quickly became able to experience and to accept both angry and admiring or even loving feelings toward me. The analysis took a decisive turn, and the material clearly

had a more powerful emotional impact on him. He subsequently reported that during the period of greatest anger he had, for the first time in the analysis, felt "really myself."

I see my departure from anonymity—a departure that with my new definition I can say promoted neutrality—as relatively minor. It also happened well into the analysis. With other patients, the more active technique must come earlier (sometimes from the first session) or be more dramatic. In contrast to Poland's assertion, my intervention did not truncate the most intense transferential feelings. In fact, the patient could not have tolerated sustained rage until after I had ventured to become less anonymous. Nor did the change in my position make things more comfortable in any conventional sense. The change enabled the patient to feel that I was not self-protective, hostile, and small-minded in the way he had experienced his father. This enhanced his sense of analytic safety, but that in turn allowed the emergence of a range of feelings that were at least temporarily more dangerous to both of us and to the continuation of the analysis than the earlier indifference had been.

Defining neutrality as optimal tension between the patient's experience of us as dangerous or safe objects gives a clear reference point *in the patient's experience* for evaluating our interventions and for monitoring our technique throughout the course of an analysis. By relying on this standard, we have a good chance of maintaining the neutral posture, which I continue to believe best serves the goals of psychoanalytic treatment.

Freud's Playground Reconsidered

TRANSFERENCE analysis, most clinicians agree, is at the core of their approach to treatment. Whereas the analyst's neutrality provides an emotional climate that makes treatment possible, transference evokes the experiences that become the focus of interpretations. Early on, Freud said that "any line of investigation" that begins with the two facts of transference and resistance "has a right to call itself psycho-analysis" (1914b, p. 16) regardless of where it might lead. More than three quarters of a century later, almost nobody disagrees. From the most conservative drive theorist to the most radical interpersonalist, and through all the intermediate shadings of orthodoxy and dissent, there is a consensus—perhaps the only one in our discipline—that ultimately psychoanalysis is transference analysis.

Because there is so little that psychoanalysts can agree about, our shared appreciation of transference has come to embody a kind of social bond: it distinguishes us a group. There are some disagreements about it, to be sure. Some believe that transference matters most when it serves as resistance to the work of analysis; others see transference phenomena as the main source of data in any analysis. Some believe that we should address transference phenomena quickly and frequently, others slowly and more cautiously. Some believe that there is a "real relationship" in the analysis, different from the transference, while others find that the distinction vitiates the power of unconscious processes. Controversy about transference fills our journals. We are united, however, by the fact that we understand the rules of transference, while nonanalysts do not.

But even that consensus masks a great deal of disagreement and, ultimately, confusion. Perhaps most strikingly, there are many different opin-

ions about what, exactly, is transferred. Is it a wish? A need, a defense, an affect, an attitude, an expectation, a perception? All of these? The assumptions that different analysts make about these possibilities are rarely articulated, and usually must be inferred from clinical discussions. When all is said and done, however, different analysts work with assumptions that are so widely disparate that they barely address the same process. This leads not only to variations in the way transference is interpreted, but to vast differences in the way the psychoanalytic situation is structured clinically and conceptualized theoretically.

Related to this, there are serious questions about what it means to "analyze" and then to "resolve" the transference. Once, early in the history of psychoanalysis, there was a clear answer to that. Today, with changed views on the phenomena that constitute transference, the meaning cannot be the same. But, because our group identity remains so tied up with transference analysis, we are stuck with the old goals.

THE FIRST psychoanalytic transference appeared in the first psychoanalytic therapy, Breuer's treatment of Anna O. Like many transferences since then, Anna's feelings for her analyst were not put into words; they were expressed through a false pregnancy that developed as the treatment was coming to an end. Breuer reacted to this unmistakable but indirect expression of passion not as an analyst but as a Victorian gentleman whose sensibilities had been offended; he withdrew from the case. It was Freud, always able to snatch theoretical victory from the jaws of therapeutic disaster, who characterized Anna's longing as an inevitable development in any psychoanalysis.

What frightened Breuer, Freud suggested, was simply a piece of his patient's past, a fragment of archaic desire that had been detached from its moorings by the probing force of analytic inquiry. Unanchored and distressing, the desire attached itself to the doctor. The patient made a "false connection" between the wish and the figure who stirred it up. Transference is the product of this false connection (Breuer and Freud, 1895, p. 302).

It is fascinating to follow Freud's thinking about transference over the twenty years following publication of *Studies on Hysteria*. He is grappling with a phenomenon that gives analysis enormous therapeutic power, but simultaneously threatens to destroy every therapeutic encounter and even the psychoanalytic movement itself. Transference is inherently and by def-

inition disruptive; whether "positive" or "negative" it sunders the presumptive safety of the patient-doctor relationship. Equally dangerous, as the news of transference spreads beyond the consulting room, questions arise in people's minds. What is going on in there? What is the (typically male) physician doing to his (typically female) patient to encourage these feelings, to entice, even to seduce?

These threats to psychoanalysis were never far from Freud's mind; they colored everything he wrote about transference. Freud was always at pains to assure his reader that the analyst does *nothing* to charm or even to influence his patient. Transference arises from the depths: "the whole readiness for these feelings is derived from elsewhere" (1916–1917, p. 442). This pronouncement was reinforced by the simultaneous evolution of Freud's drive model, with its assumption that all experience arises as a transformation of endogenous need. Transference, which Freud considered the best proof of his drive theory, was a case in point of how powerful these needs can be. Even a doctor becomes a lover under the pressure of need—consider what Anna O. made of the irreproachable Breuer.

In "The Dynamics of Transference" Freud spelled out his understanding of the origin of the patient's feeling for the doctor. Everybody, he writes, "has acquired a specific method of his own in his conduct of his erotic life—that is, in the preconditions to falling in love which he lays down, in the instincts he satisfies and the aims he sets himself in the course of it" (1912a, p. 99). It is this "conduct of his erotic life" that the patient transfers. He does so because it has been stirred up by the analytic process. Excavation leads to false connections. In *Introductory Lectures* Freud tells us that he has "unwillingly" recognized that transference appears "under the most unfavourable conditions and where there are positively grotesque incongruities, even in elderly women and in relation to grey-bearded men, even where, in our judgement, there is nothing of any kind to entice" (1916–17, p. 442). Transference, then, is the wishful direction of erotic impulses toward the unwitting, even unwilling analyst.

Strikingly, perhaps unfortunately, Freud had little new to say about transference after 1917. So his perspective was not altered by the radical changes in his clinical and theoretical formulations that came later. Transference remained anchored in the drive theory, untouched by the structural model, ideas of danger situations and safety, the more sophisticated vision of the development of object relations, or the revised affect theory. This early vision continued to make itself felt in psychoanalysis for many

years: the definition in LaPlanche and Pontalis' dictionary of psychoanalytic concepts begins with the idea that transference is "a process of actualisation of unconscious wishes" (1973, p. 455).

The assumption that transference is essentially a vicissitude of the patient's libidinal impulses, although still strongly held in some psychoanalytic circles, does not stand up well to contemporary clinical experience. As we have learned more and as theory has evolved, many analysts have become increasingly sensitive to the psychodynamic importance of defenses, object relations, danger situations, and ego capacities of various degrees of autonomy from the drives. This new awareness changed most analysts' sense of the *content* of transference. Few analysts these days would agree that transference expresses exclusively or even principally the patient's "conduct of his erotic life."

Within more or less orthodox psychoanalytic circles, change began with the work of Anna Freud. Cautiously integrating some of Wilhelm Reich's ideas into the framework of a developing ego psychology, she distinguished what she called "transference of defense" from the "transference of libidinal impulse" of Freud's original formulations. Transference of defense does not involve a wish directed toward the analyst—instead it expresses an attitude. And this transferential attitude tends to be egosyntonic. Anna Freud gives two examples of transference of defense: the patient may be moved to flee from the analyst, or the patient may submit passively. In either case the reaction depends on a particular understanding of what is going on, and it is based in the patient's perception, judgment, and reality testing. No matter what defensive posture the patient adopts, he feels that his reaction is justified by the circumstances.

In addition, Anna Freud discussed a subspecies of transference, externalizations, which she believed should be kept conceptually separate from transference proper. Externalizations do not represent repeated childhood relationships; they arise when one side of a conflict is projected onto the analyst. The patient may, for example, feel some kind of intense longing and see the analyst as hostile to it, or he himself may experience the analyst as seductive while holding on to the rejecting feelings. The concept of externalizations broadens not only our understanding of the content of transference experience, but also the way we conceptualize their source. The externalized transferences do not originate in childhood; they are adult attitudes that are felt to derive from something that is actually going on in the analysis.

Anna Freud's distinction between externalizations, defense transference,

and libidinal transference parallels the movement within psychoanalysis from an id psychology to an ego psychology in general. For over fifty years, many analysts have shifted their focus from Freud's original transference of impulse to what I suggest we call *transference of conviction*. In transference of impulse, the analyst comes alive for the patient mainly as an object of desire. In contrast, transference of conviction revolves around the patient's ideas about the analyst—his perceptions, beliefs, hunches, and hypotheses.

There are two reasons that psychoanalytic interest has shifted from transference of impulse to transference of conviction. The first is empirical, if difficult to demonstrate. Overt expressions of sexual interest are rather less frequent these days than they were in Freud's time; Sandler, Dare, and Holder suggest that "in the course of time psychoanalysts have not come to expect their patients to fall in love with them so frequently and to such a degree" (1973, p. 51). This may have to do with the cultural impact that psychoanalysis itself has had; we see few patients who don't have the idea that they are supposed to fall in love with or become sexually enthralled by their analyst. There are no hard data I know of about how many analyses begin with patients telling their analysts "I'm not going to" feel such and such—but I suspect it happens quite frequently. Patients are wary of the passions they assume we expect them to feel for us.

The second, more important, reason for the shift has less to do with what patients say than with the way analysts interpret what they hear. Viewed from this perspective, transference of conviction and transference of impulse are not different phenomena but alternative ways of understanding what is going on. Freud of course always believed that the impulse drives the conviction: in more formal theoretical terms we would say that transformations of the wish determine the experiential characteristics of the object relation. The patient's transferential conviction, then, functions mainly as a clue to the underlying transference wish. The conviction is superficial, preconscious, defensive. Analysis depends on moving beyond the conviction to its "deeper" wishful determinants.

In contrast, many contemporary theorists believe that the impulse arises out of the conviction. This reverses the direction of analytic inquiry. Even faced with an openly expressed erotic wish, the analyst would want to uncover the experiential context—the conviction—from which the wish was born. The wish itself is a clue to the underlying transferential impression. Weiss, Sampson, and their colleagues are explicit about this way of construing events in the transference: "a patient may invite the analyst to

reciprocate his professed love to test his unconscious belief that if he were sexual or affectionate toward a parental figure, he would seduce him" (1986, p. 269). I would take it a step further: the sexual demand itself may grow out of the patient's belief that there is something seductive about the analyst or the analytic situation. If that kind of belief seems unlikely and distorted on its face, recall that the possibility occurred to Freud almost as soon as he began working psychoanalytically. In *Studies on Hysteria* he discusses the possibility of treatment becoming disrupted when the patient fears "becoming sexually dependent" on the analyst. This is likely to occur because of the "special solicitude inherent in the treatment" (Breuer and Freud, 1895, p. 302). Unfortunately, Freud did not carry this early insight into his later formulations of transference.

Despite many contemporary analysts' tendency to hear convictions rather than impulses in their patients' transferences, the concept itself remains burdened by its origins. Perhaps the most important consequence of this is that our method of analyzing transference and the goals of transference analysis remains rooted in Freud's early formulations. It is important to begin disentangling some of this archaic residue from what remains clinically and theoretically vital.

Distortion or Creation?

When Freud created the concept of transference of impulse, it was easy to assume that the impulse itself was contextually inappropriate and that any impressions that the patient might construct as rationales were based on misunderstandings. This presumption could be justified on both metapsychological and clinical grounds. Metapsychologically, all wishes were presumed to originate with the purely endogenous stirrings of libido and were thought to be given their particular ideational form according to the patient's infantile history of satisfactions and frustrations. Thus neither the occurrence of desire nor the imagined circumstances of its fulfillment reflected the realities of the psychoanalytic situation. Clinically, the extravagant claim on the analyst's time, not to mention his libido, that is implied by the erotic demand makes it easy to believe that any transference of impulse is distorted.

It is much more difficult to presume distortion when we are dealing with transference of conviction. Convictions are complex cognitive constructions that are never determined purely imaginatively any more than they are ever naive renderings of external reality. Irwin Hoffman has said

that we cannot deny "that there is any aspect of the patient's experience that pertains to the therapist's inner motives that can be unequivocally designated as distorting of reality. Similarly [we cannot deny] that there is any aspect of this experience that can be unequivocally designated as faithful to reality" (1983, p. 394).

Yet we still find transference-as-distortion, a relic of the origins of the concept. Greenson, for example, despite a broadened vision of the content of transference that includes conviction, writes, "Transference reactions are always inappropriate . . . The transference reaction is unsuitable in its current context; but it was once an appropriate reaction to a past situation" (1967, p. 152). In a similar vein, Sandler, Dare, and Holder define transference as "*a specific illusion* which develops in regard to the other person, one which, unbeknown to the subject, represents, in some of its features, a repetition of a relationship towards an important figure in the person's past" (1973, p. 47). The key word here is "illusion." An illusion is experienced very much like the kind of conviction I have described. At the same time, it is a mistaken conviction, a belief that has been floating around in the patient's unconscious forever, awaiting only the appearance of appropriate conditions for attaching itself to some indifferent object.

The emphasis on distortion can be found even in the formulations of radical thinkers operating within the relational model. Consider Sullivan's concept of parataxic distortion, the rough equivalent of transference; consider, in fact, the very term. Sullivan defines parataxis as follows: "The characteristics of a person that would be agreed to by a large number of competent observers may not appear to you to be the characteristics of the person toward whom you are making adjustive or maladjustive movements. The *real* characteristics of the other fellow at that time may be of negligible importance to the interpersonal situation" (1954, p. 25).

The implications of seeing transference as distortion play out clearly in a vignette given by Otto Kernberg. It is a nice example because it is apparently hypothetical and can therefore be discussed without accusing the author of being crippled by countertransferentially based blindspots and without implications that the analyst has mishandled the treatment.

> Let's assume that I have a hole in my sock, and my patient becomes enraged. Why? He doesn't know. He is just enraged that I should have a hole in my sock. I ask him: "What are you so angry about?" The patient has to think, starts rationalizing, and after we analyze his effort to find some rational explanation for something essentially irrational, it turns out that it reminds him of his mother with holes in her stockings, of her neglectful attitude, of the

sloppy attitude of his mother. *Now this is for me a transference reaction* . . . It is, first of all, an inappropriate affect and, by the same token, the enactment of an object relation (1987, p. 124, my italics).

Kernberg's description of his patient's reaction is a clear case of transference of conviction. Nowhere in his example does he suggest that the patient's reaction either defends against or is driven by any underlying wish. But he concludes that the reaction is transferential on two grounds: the intensity of the patient's anger and the similarity of his conviction about Kernberg to an important but evidently inattended conviction about his mother. The emotional magnitude registers on a kind of seismic instrument that alerts the analyst to a disturbance of something somewhere, and the parallel memory of the mother explains why the patient should think such things about his analyst.

What should occur to any analyst working within the framework of transference of conviction is that the patient is not *simply* repeating an object relation and that his affect is not *simply* inappropriate. Rather, he is expressing something that he believes to be true about his analyst. He is not simply repeating the relationship with his neglectful mother—he is asserting and reacting to a perception that Kernberg is *in fact* like his mother. This would have to raise questions about what has happened in the analysis to give the patient that impression. I doubt that the hole in Kernberg's sock is enough. Seeing the hole has a special poignance for this patient because it reflects something deeper about the patient's analytic experience. One would certainly want to know more about that. And perhaps one would even want to know how Kernberg came to have such an obvious hole in his sock in the first place. Such questions are not likely to come up in this analysis, however, because the inquiry has been diverted from the misperceived present to the etiologically crucial past.

Let me stress that the kinds of convictions that become activated in the transference are not merely "objective" reproductions of people or of events. Neither are they consensually validated narratives or versions of what has happened; it is often difficult to describe convictions meaningfully, much less to arrive at agreement about them with others. Instead I see them as deeply personal constructions that reflect the person's wishes, needs, hopes, fears, memories, perceptions, and anticipations. Convictions, like all representations, are the product of creative acts, which give shape to the world in which we live.

Accordingly, transference of conviction does not *pervert* meaning, it

creates meaning; our convictions make *a* life *our* life. The traditional dichotomy of a "correctly perceived" real relationship and a "distorted" transference relationship is virtually irrelevant within the framework of transference of conviction. The distinction between what is real and what is distorted fades when we think of creative acts.

In a lovely essay about the day his glasses broke, the near-blind James Thurber wrote about the richness that can come from not seeing clearly:

> I saw the Cuban flag flying over a national bank, I saw a gay old lady with a gray parasol walk right through the side of a truck, I saw a cat roll across a street in a small striped barrel, I saw bridges rise lazily into the air, like balloons . . .
>
> With perfect vision, one is inextricably trapped in the workaday world, a prisoner of reality . . . lost in the commonplace of America . . . For the hawk-eyed person life has none of those soft edges which for me blur into fantasy" (1936, pp. 241–242).

Breaking his glasses left Thurber not misperceiving but perceiving differently. Compare the idea of the critic Harold Bloom that the creativity of the major western poets depends on what he calls their distortion of the vision of their predecessors, a distortion that makes way for their own particular sensibility (Bloom, 1973). For both Thurber and Bloom, creativity grows from a dialectic between a kind of perceptual clarity and a more deeply idiosyncratic perspective; in the final analysis, creative living depends on the ability to trust and enjoy what you see rather than on bringing what you see up to a particular level of accuracy.

There are relatively few psychoanalysts of any theoretical persuasion who share an appreciation of the creative potential inherent in the human capacity for constructing representations and, ultimately, for transference. One of the few who does is Hans Loewald, who says that what is transferred is "the intensity of the unconscious, of the infantile ways of experiencing life that have no language and little organization, but [that do have] the indestructibility and power of the origins of life," and that "without such transference, or to the extent to which such transference miscarries, human life becomes sterile and an empty shell" (1960, p. 250).

The Resolution of Transference

Both the goal and the method of transference analysis rest on the idea that transference arises when unconscious wishes interfere with accurate per-

ception. In his paper on the theory of psychoanalytic technique, James Strachey distinguished two stages in the construction of a "mutative" interpretation. First the analyst reacts in a way that establishes himself as different from the patient's archaic bad objects; he thereby becomes introjected into the patient's inner world as a benign superego. He is more tolerant of previously forbidden impulses than other people in the patient's life were or than the patient himself has come to be. Then, having become the transferential target of these same impulses, he works toward explaining them, locating them in the patient's prehistory. Strachey put it this way: "at the critical moment of the emergence into consciousness of the released quantity of id-energy [the patient must be able] to distinguish between his phantasy object and the real analyst" (1934, p. 146).

While Strachey emphasized characteristics of the analytic object relationship far more than anyone had previously, his two stages of the mutative interpretation parallel the process of transference analysis that Freud described. First we establish the conditions within which the transference can emerge—the analytic frame—and then we "work through" the transference manifestations, aiming ultimately at their resolution. We create a situation that makes it possible for the patient to attempt "to put his passions into action," and then we "compel him to fit these emotional impulses into the nexus of the treatment and of his life history" (1912a, p. 108). Years later, Freud described the same process by arguing, "The transference is made conscious to the patient by the analyst, and it is resolved by convincing him that in his transference-attitude he is *re-experiencing* emotional relations which had their origin in his earliest object-attachments during the repressed period of his childhood" (1925b, p. 43).

There is a striking difference in the emotional tone that underlies these two steps in the analysis of transference. The first step—very much like the establishment of a neutral atmosphere as I've described it—requires attention to the patient's anxiety about sharing or even becoming aware of thoughts that are ignored in conventional circumstances. Consider the sorts of things that occur to us, fleetingly, in the courses of any intimate relationship. Sexual impulses in all their genital and pregenital forms, hostile fantasies of murder and mutilation, intense envy and jealousy, insights into the carefully guarded secrets of the other person—any of these may occur to us, but we will turn away quickly or divert them into more socially acceptable forms. Revealing our tranference requires that we catch

these transient thoughts, dwell on them, and describe them in detail to the very person who is their object.

Both Freud and Strachey recognized the emotional difficulty of doing this. Although neither of them was quite explicit about it, each acknowledged that becoming aware of the transference required a great risk on the patient's part. Freud (1912a) stressed that the patient's ability to take this risk depended on the "unobjectionable positive transference"—the preformed attitudes toward the physician and toward the possibility of cure itself that motivated the patient to seek treatment in the first place. Strachey, more impressed by interpersonal nuance, saw the analyst's behavior, his analytic attitude, as the key factor. However we understand the details, there is consensus that to come to know transference requires that the patient feel safe enough to venture beyond the usual boundaries of awareness. Thus the emotional tone of the first stage of the analysis of transference involves the patient's feeling of comfort.

In contrast, the second phase, the resolution of the transference, has a confrontational tone. Freud says that the patient must be "convinced" that his feelings are inappropriate to the contemporary situation and "compelled" to relocate his impulses to the archaic past. Even Strachey suggests that the process depends on the patient's ability to give up his conviction of the reality of his feelings. If the first stage of interpretation focuses on facilitating the patient's capacity to *share* his experience, the second stage is occupied with getting him to *renounce* that same experience.

THIS vision of the analysis and resolution of the transference may make some sense if we assume that the content of transference consists of wishful impulses. The patient's erotic life has been fixated at or has regressed to infantile strivings; he is left repeatedly pursuing less than adult goals with unsuitable or unavailable people. Only if his libido is freed from its archaic aims and objects will the patient be able to pursue mature goals; only then will he be able to achieve real as opposed to imaginary and therefore incomplete satisfaction.

Accordingly, we would want to "convince" the patient to give up his transference. Doing so will free him from a regressive trap and allow him to enjoy an unfettered genitality. Renouncing his transferential claims on the analyst allows him to initiate and to maintain both raw and aim-inhibited sexual relationships with appropriate, available, extrafamilial partners. Further, since cognitive distortions within the transference are

secondary to the patient's conflicted attempts to make the analyst into a libidinal object, these are bound to be dissolved along with the renunciation of the transference wishes. This permits the patient to have a "realistic" vision of the analyst. He will be able to see the analyst for what he really is and to appreciate both the possibilities and the limitations of the analytic relationship.

The transference is considered analyzed, and the analysis itself is considered complete, when these goals have been achieved. If we think in terms of transference of impulse, the goal of transference resolution affirms the patient's claim to take his rightful place in the adult world. But what might it mean to "resolve" transference of conviction? Because our vision of transference resolution has not changed along with the shifting sensibility about the content of transference, we are left with an anomalous situation. Resolving transference of conviction along the lines of the traditional model would require the patient to give up a particular set of beliefs about the analyst. These beliefs are deeply felt and ego-syntonic (Sandler, Dare, and Holder, 1973), and even from an outsider's perspective they are plausible versions of what is going on (Gill, 1982; Hoffman, 1983). Beyond that, they can sharpen the patient's awareness of particular facets of the analyst's personality, and they open the door to awareness of his own creative vision.

Consider a brief example. A female patient, scanning my office, asked the question—reasonable in the circumstances—"Why is it that the only color you've ever heard of is brown?" I was initially taken aback by the question; it was not one to which I had given a great deal of thought. After a pause, I decided to ask her why she believed that I would know more about that than she did. The question confused her at first, but when she realized that I meant it seriously she began speculating. She is a perceptive person, and once she got into it she found that she had quite a lot to say. I had a range of reactions to what she came up with—some of it seemed quite accurate, some seemed plausible, some rather dubious. But I want to stress two things. First, all of what she said was colored by her somewhat eccentric, often troubled and troubling way of looking at things. Second, though I found all of it interesting, I doubt that any of it would have occurred to me spontaneously.

Significant aspects of this woman's transference were contained in the convictions that emerged in these speculations about my taste in colors. What in this transference must she be "convinced" is incorrect or "compelled" to renounce? Which of her convictions about me could I even say,

in all fairness, were wrong? Do I know better? I'm not sure, but I can say that in this instance I found the patient's speculations more interesting and illuminating than my own. When we shift our attention from impulse to conviction we pull the rug out from under our comfortable notions of what we should be doing with the transference. There is quite a difference between discarding an unsatisfiable wish and abandoning a way of seeing the world.

The representational model that I have proposed lends itself well to conceptualizing the goal and method of analyzing transference of conviction. These transferences reflect the influence of evoked events and their multilayered re-representations on the patient's impressions of the analyst. As the analyst's neutrality increases the flexibility of the dominant self representation, an increasingly greater range of re-representations becomes accessible to consciousness. At this point the interpretive activity of the analyst takes center stage. The analyst tries to articulate the emerging representations, locating elements of the current transference experience that make them vivid for the patient. The goal is not to confirm or disconfirm anything that the patient believes; the analyst's interest is in facilitating the patient's awareness of the range and richness of her experience.

I will illustrate this process by describing the sequential emergence of four transference paradigms in the analysis of a young businessman, L. This view is necessarily panoramic—I'm describing the flow of a lengthy analysis. Each paradigm involves a number of individual convictions; the transference feelings emerged before L. could have put the convictions themselves into words. I would describe the first paradigm as adaptive. L. saw me as interested in doing a good job, attentive to him in a professional sort of way, having an interesting slant on life, somewhat aloof, perhaps more skeptical about him than I was letting on. In response he was polite and acquiescent, notably easy to get along with, rather bland in manner. He respected my privacy and honored what he had heard was the rule of analytic anonymity. He didn't challenge me, although I frequently sensed a kind of cautious passivity that worked to deflect our more emotionally intense exchanges.

As L. became more involved in the analysis, a second transference paradigm emerged, one that can be called paranoid (although I mean this in a dynamic and by no means diagnostic sense). This deepened his initial vision of me as reserved and skeptical. He saw me as out to trip him up, to catch him in moments of ambition, competitiveness, or hostility. This he saw as my perogative, the reason I had chosen such a powerful profes-

sion in the first place. Needless to say, it gave new meaning to his own caution and politeness, as his ways of hiding from a deeply feared, always dangerous adversary. They also provided effective cover through which he could scrutinize me, searchingly, to assess how prone to attack I might be on a given day.

Gradually a third possibility developed. The balance of strength shifted and L. began to see himself as stronger and even dangerous to me. I think of this transference as following manic-depressive lines, again speaking only dynamically. It began to occur to L. that he was younger than I am, that much in life that he could look forward to I could only look back on. His work in the business world, which earlier had seemed degraded in contrast to the altruistic, intellectually and morally virtuous work of an analyst, had a different feel. He was active in the world of men, powerful, a mover and shaker. But I sat around worrying about peoples' worries; it was woman's work at best, a kind of silly way for a grown-up to spend his time. The affective tone surrounding these thoughts varied considerably. At some times he was thrilled to recognize that he liked what he had, and even that he liked having what I did not. At other times he was genuinely mortified to think how damaged and weakened I must feel by his success and by the comparisons he was making. I must hate him for it but, even more, I must hate myself.

The final paradigm that emerged is one I will call "excited." Now he saw me as an attractive and appealing person who could also be attracted to him. We were, he realized, men together—perhaps it's more accurate to say that we were boys together. Although we each had our separate lives to lead, there was also something that we shared; we met together in a special and emotionally powerful way. There was a distinctly erotic charge to the sessions, an excitement that he could be shy about, frightened of, and even occasionally enjoy. He was able to think, tentatively at first and then with more constancy, that I could enjoy and even be excited about him.

As we were able to get to know his transferences, L.'s vision of me became increasingly lively, subtle, and textured. I became, uniquely, *his* analyst. Each paradigm elaborated different impressions that L. had of me. With L., as with many patients, I came to know a version of myself that I had never known before, or never known in quite that way. L.'s tranference enriched my experience of myself. But even if it hadn't—even in the unlikely event that I'd heard it all before—the gradual unfolding of these transferences is what gave life to me for L.

But alongside its creative potential, the human capacity for transferences embodies our most debilitating tendencies as well. Why? I would suggest that each transference paradigm, for all that it reveals, is also defensive: while each gives birth to some possibilities, each simultaneously restricts others. L.'s "adaptive" version of me warded off more intense paranoid, manic, depressive, and excited feelings. The paranoia warded off guilt, the excitement defended against paranoia—each, when L. initially experienced it, seemed inevitable and so limited the range of his experience. Each dictated an inevitable version of me that, however much it promoted creative insight, closed off other possibilities. Transference can be optimally creative only when the patient can be playful with it—only, that is, when he can experience any particular reaction as reflecting but one part of a vast range of possibilities. This depends on the freedom to be aware of as many transference paradigms as possible. The process is similar to what I have discussed as the capacity to experience previously repressed re-representations; the description points the way to what I think of as the genuinely therapeutic analysis of transference.

Along these lines, let me stress that while L.'s various transferences did emerge successively, the earlier paradigms did not disappear as new ones were elaborated. Just as representations last forever, patients never really renounce particular patterns of conviction—they are not (and should not be) resolved in the classical sense. There were times even at the very end of his long analysis when L., having experienced me as excited about him, would dissect my motives in an effort to find anger, competitiveness, and so on. This might in turn yield to the earlier politeness and acquiescence, with their underlying convictions about me.

Furthermore, although new transference paradigms do emerge as analysis proceeds, I don't think that what is therapeutic is that a "less realistic" paradigm yields to one that is "more realistic." This, again, would be the version of things in the classic model of transference resolution. But who is to judge which of the paradigms is realistic, especially at any given time? Indeed, I am convinced that each of the paradigms evoked in the course of L.'s analysis gave him insight into something important about me, as well as into something important about himself. Each version revealed different convictions that L. had about himself and about me; each enabled him to become conscious of something about me that he would have repressed under the sway of the other transferences.

I think that if any transference paradigm did disappear, the patient's creative range would be compromised. L.'s potential for depressive guilt

sensitized him to people's capacity to envy him for his abilities and achievements. "Resolving" this transference—renouncing it as a misdirected erotic demand might be renounced—would have returned L. to where he was before the analysis had facilitated his capacity to risk awareness of that particular transference paradigm. He might, for instance, have reverted to the manifest blandness that characterized his adaptive presentation of himself. The effect of our work together was not that L. lost his depressive convictions, or any others, but that he became able to experience each conviction as merely one of many components of his repertoire.

It was also important for L. to understand what might have triggered the shift from one paradigm to another. These shifts typically follow experiences of anxiety that arise in response to something the patient feels toward or notices about the analyst. In becoming increasingly able to catch these moments of transition, the patient learns about the defensive function of his transference convictions, and becomes more and more able to free himself from compulsive attachment to any one. This expands the limits of his creativity and perceptiveness, limits determined by the accessibility of all the various transference paradigms.

When they reveal their transferences, our patients give us access to their most personal ways of constructing and living in the world. The various transferences differ in terms of how comfortable they are to the patient. Some, like L.'s adaptive transference and to a lesser extent his paranoia, feel more familiar. These less jealously guarded ways of creating experience become the first transference paradigms to emerge in the analysis: they are enacted quickly and may even be put into words and openly discussed.

Other paradigms—L.'s manic-depressive and excited transferences are examples—are among the most subjectively tender contents of mental life. Both the self and the object experiences that get actualized in these transferences are sources of deeply felt shame and humiliation. Further, they facilitate insights into the analyst that arouse profound feelings of guilt. Resistance to the emergence of these transference paradigms is motivated both by fears of revealing a contemptible side of the self and by protective feelings directed toward the analyst.

Other analysts—most notably Merton Gill—have stressed the idea that transference analysis moves the patient from a sense of inevitability about his experience toward increasing flexibility. But even Gill stresses that flexibility comes from showing the patient that his experience of the analyst, while plausible, is significantly determined by his archaic past. To me that

suggests that while the experience may be understandable it is fundamentally inappropriate, or at least slightly off.

Certainly I agree that part of what works in transference analysis is that the patient learns what has happened in his life to give his convictions their particular shape. It is also important for the patient to learn that convictions in general—his own and perhaps also the analyst's—are significantly determined by prior experience, belief systems, needs, and desires. This is the clinical lesson of the idea that all mental contents are multiply determined personal constructions. But ultimately the patient's ability to use the transference creatively depends on his awareness that he himself has other ways of experiencing the analyst and that these are warded off by the "inevitable" convictions. It is in taking the risks that reveal the intricate tapestry of our transference convictions—unveiling how we make the world tick—that we get to know ourselves and allow others to know us. That is the analytic goal, and that is why we work so hard to promote and deepen our patients' awareness of their transference.

The Analyst's Countertransference

Tranference of conviction stirs up powerful resistances. Despite conventional psychoanalytic wisdom, it often arouses less anxiety to acknowledge impulses than to acknowledge perceptions. This is especially true when the object of the convictions is present; patients have an easier time describing their analysts to their friends than to the analyst himself.

One angry but perceptive patient gave dramatic expression to the anxiety she felt about putting her impressions into words. She had spent a good part of her session drawing a portrait of me which contained significant amounts of vitriol and uncomfortably accurate observation. When she was finished she hesitated, seemed somewhat abashed, and said, "Well of course if I didn't know it was all projection, I couldn't have said a word of it."

Why should expressing convictions be so difficult? Although it is a question with many answers, a naive observer would be at least partly correct if he suggested that our patients don't fully believe us when we tell them that they can say anything that comes to mind. They seem especially skeptical when it comes to talking about what they see in us. It is as if they are afraid that what they have to say about us could potentially destroy the analyst as a benign presence.

The situation recalls a comment of Hartmann's. As he was becoming more attuned to the interpersonal determinants of developmental experience, he wrote, "What the mother . . . is 'neurotically' afraid of can . . . mean 'real' danger for the child" (1956, p. 258). Similarly, the analyst's vulnerability to his patient's convictions can create a realistic danger within the analysis. The patient unconsciously senses the analyst's anxiety and fears that what he observes may threaten the analyst's sense of well-being. The patient, in turn, feels endangered, leading him to stifle his perceptions and to renounce his creative potential and even his reality testing.

Hoffman (1983) has pointed out a form of resistance that is well suited to deal with the dangers posed by the awareness of transference of conviction. The patient, he suggests, may tenaciously hold on to a belief that the analyst is in fact the blank screen that theory prescribes he should be. In a striking example of this, I worked once with a young man who was a personnel director. His job required him to form quick impressions about people and make judgments about how they would fit in various positions. Because of the nature of the work involved, the decisions were based more on the applicant's personality than on the level or type of skill. For two years in therapy this man insisted that he saw nothing in me to allow him to form any opinion about me whatsoever.

Still there is a great deal for any patient to observe in the psychoanalytic situation from the very beginning. The patient, entering the analyst's office for the first time and meeting the person in whom he has invested a wide range of hopes and fears, carefully scans the environment for clues about what he can expect. Needless to say, he finds a great deal. He sees a person of a certain age, social class, sex, and style, someone who meets him in a particular way. And immediately he begins to draw conclusions.

The conclusions that patients draw can be disturbing to everyone involved. Although psychoanalytic writings tend to stress the patient's reaction to the analyst's power, status, and authority, there is another side to that coin. Consider a few commonplace examples. A young patient with an older analyst must deal with what it means to be stronger and more vigorous than his analyst, or to have a more active and varied sex life, or simply to have more years to live. On a number of occasions I have worked with female patients who had previous treatment with women whom they knew to be unmarried and childless. These patients typically could not bring up their own social or sexual or marital satisfactions and dreams in a fully unrestrained way; they were afraid of touching too closely on what

they knew must be issues with which the analyst had struggled and suffered. One man who had a net worth of several million dollars had every reason to assume that my own net worth was considerably less. He was someone who worked hard for his financial success but who was so guilt-ridden about it that he dressed like a workman. It was a long time before he was able to express an emotion like gleefulness about having more money than I did. Another patient, a younger man, didn't have a great deal of money when he entered analysis, but he fully intended to. He rarely allowed himself to talk about his plans, especially with any sense of eager anticipation, because he was fearful of expressing enthusiasm about his real potential of surpassing me financially.

As analysis proceeds, the opportunities for the patient to make uncomfortable observations multiply. How, for example, will a patient who is optimistic by virtue of temperament and life circumstances react to her perception that her analyst has reached a stage of life where he is resigned to his personal limitations? Or, for that matter, to the depressive style that characterizes at least a few analysts? How will the intellectually gifted and ambitious patient respond to an analyst who is also ambitious but less talented? These sorts of situations remind me of Therese Benedek's comment that "sooner or later, the therapist may stamp the patient's attitude, his empathy, his guessing the truth as 'provocative behavior'" (1949, p. 497).

Benedek saw the analyst's potential vulnerability to the patient's transferential convictions. These convictions can have special power: they are frequently astute, and they are dramatically elaborated because of the intense emotions evoked by the treatment process. The developing relationship with the analyst is precisely the kind of situation that will evoke a wide range of repressed events and associated re-representations. These color the immediate experience, strengthening the already highly charged impressions and beliefs. Ogden (1989) graphically depicts the primitive anxieties that emerge—much disguised—even in the first analytic hour. In sharp contrast, Weiss, Sampson, and their colleagues (1986) describe the way the analyst, again from the very beginning, is a repository for the patient's fondest hopes. Despite vastly different sensibilities, both formulations address the evocative potential even of the initial contact, and its power to generate intense (and perhaps troubling) convictions about the analyst. From the start the analyst is exposed to a patient who holds a specific image of him, based on what the patient has noticed but has also intensely elaborated.

A clinical approach that directs attention toward the transference of impulse can serve as a protective shield for the analyst. Arlow, for one, is able to distance himself from his patients' observations because he believes that "transference may be understood as representing how the individual misperceives, misinterprets, and misresponds to, the data of perception, in terms of the mental set created by persistent unconscious fantasies" (1985a, p. 526). The customer is always wrong, and the analyst can safely interpret the wish that lies behind the patient's distorted vision.

Consider a simple example. When the patient says to his analyst "I think you're angry with me," the analyst is likely to look for and to find a conflicted wish that underlies the comment. Perhaps the thought derives from projection of the patient's own angry impulse, or it may express a longed-for masochistic submission, or it may embody anxiety-driven ideas about retaliation for libidinal interest in the analyst. The content of the wish does not affect my example. What matters is the premise that analytic leverage depends on uncovering the wishful origins of the putative observation. Paying attention to the patient's conviction would arrest the analytic process at a superficial level.

This approach ignores the perceptual basis of the patient's impression and focuses attention on what he fears most in himself. We interpret the impulse in its most elemental, least sublimated form, and we give short shrift to the conviction from which the impulse arises. There are opportunities to be self-protective at every turn. When the patient talks about ambition, we may hear thinly veiled murderous aims; when he wants something for himself, we think in terms of envy-driven impulses to destroy what the analyst has. When the patient challenges our sense of self in some frightening way, drive theory can work to decrease our feelings of vulnerability and anxiety, at the expense of increasing our tendency to engage in and rationalize countertransferential acting out.

Two brief clinical examples will illustrate this self-protectiveness, both drawn from cases I supervised. In the first the problems were serious enough that the analyst's insistent interpretations of the patient's impulses constituted a genuine, intractable acting out. As a result the analysis had a negative impact on the patient. The second, and more typical, example is from the work of a particularly talented and thoughtful analyst. This treatment had beneficial results.

In the first example, the patient, on the eve of a professional public appearance that constituted both recognition of his abilities and an opportunity to further his career, had a series of dreams in which he was

responsible for the deaths of older men and women who had been his mentors. The analyst, who appeared to me somewhat frustrated about his own level of professional achievement, was quick to interpret the patient's feeling that his ambition was tantamount to murder. The patient, who as I see it had the dream in the first place largely because he feared how his ambition and achievement would be experienced by others, was quick to accept the interpretation because it neatly reestablished a comfortable neurotic balance. The analyst, after the interpretation, appeared unthreatened by what the patient was up to; in fact he seemed strong in his ability to name the patient's hateful, homicidal impulses. And the patient saw himself as bad, in a way that had become familiar to him. He escaped the sense of himself as challenging to the rather uncertain and frustrated people with whom he had grown up, and to the analyst with whom the earlier circumstances had been recreated.

Nothing in what I have just said should be taken to deny that the patient wished to defeat and even to destroy his mentors, his parents, or, most especially, his analyst. People tend to want to do such things, and these aims mingle with motives organized around ambition, achievement, separation-individuation, assertiveness, self-cohesion or whatever. I would suggest, however, that the analyst's premature interpretation of these aims was an expression of his own countertransferential reactions not only to the patient's competitiveness but also to his success. Interpreting the impulse too quickly stirred the patient's guilt, shame, and anxiety, making it impossible for him to appreciate his convictions about the impact that his ambitions and achievements would have on the analyst. In this situation, analytic progress depended on the patient learning in some way not only that he *wanted* to harm the analyst but that he *believed* he was at risk of doing so.

The second patient was a man in his thirties who entered analysis because of a chronic passivity that he felt limited both his professional development and the satisfaction he was able to get out of relationships with women. He was one of three children, the only son of a successful small-town physician. The father, despite constraints on his time and a characterological preoccupation with his work, apparently had a good deal to offer his son emotionally, but there were strings attached. These essentially involved demands that his son participate in activities that were of interest to the father and that he participate on the father's time schedule.

The analyst was an unusually dynamic and quite ambitious man. These characteristics were apparent despite his equally evident gentleness and

sensitivity. He and the patient had developed a relationship that was very positive, both in terms of the tone of the transference and also in terms of its collaborative elements. At the time I am discussing, the analyst had canceled one session a week for three straight weeks in order to attend a series of professional meetings. Not incidentally, these encompassed a range of interests and involved organizations in which the analyst played a leadership role.

The patient's response to the analyst's comings and goings was interesting. He talked at length about his reactions to the canceled appointments, addressing mainly a feeling of longing for the analyst and disappointment over what he would be missing. Characteristically, he was forthcoming in his associations, which involved a textured range of feelings that were interpretable in terms of the pleasure and security he experienced in the analysis, and in terms of angry feelings about being deprived of these. The picture that emerged was a consistent one: the patient needed the analyst and analysis, which he experienced as gratifying a range of dependent and more or less sublimated homosexual impulses.

There was just one fly in the ointment of the analysis of this man's reaction to the disruption of treatment: he offered no speculation about what the analyst was up to, except for an unusually bland rationalization that maybe he was doing it purposely, to provoke some movement toward independence. From my perspective, this unreflective and unlikely hypothesis of the patient's was strikingly devoid of his usual psychological sophistication. Equally intriguing, because it was equally uncharacteristic, was the analyst's failure to inquire further into the patient's fantasy or even to notice what was missing in his version of the disruption. It seemed fine with him to let well enough alone and to accept that the patient's experience of his absence could best be conceptualized in terms of thwarted needs and of his frustrated and angry reaction to the deprivation.

Had the patient seen something in the analyst, perhaps something to which he was especially sensitive because of his relationship with his father? Had he also assumed that, like his father, the analyst would neither encourage nor even tolerate the mention of whatever had been noticed? And was there some truth in this—were there aspects of the situation that the analyst found uncomfortable? Pursuing this line of inquiry in supervision uncovered a range of relevant thoughts. The analyst felt guilty about leaving both his patients and his family; he questioned whether his ambitions were interfering with his more personal involvements and preferred at least for the moment not to dwell on the conflict. Further, he

wondered whether this kind of career goal interfered which what he "owed" his patients, and he was even more generally concerned about whether it reflected adversely on what he was prepared to offer others. In short, although he could not have articulated it in advance of our discussion, he was worried about whether he was like his patient's father in ways that violated his sense of what he thought other people deserved from him.

Without supervision, this analysis would have remained at the level of impulse and of the patient's conflicts about his neediness. More insidiously, it would have recreated in the patient's experience the pattern of fitting himself into the schedule and vulnerabilities of the analyst/father, never allowing himself the freedom to challenge the situation. Analysis would have perpetuated his feeling that he was childish, tied dependently and homosexually to a man who had much to give but whose behavior could not be questioned.

It is my impression that many analyses, including some superficially beneficial ones, have concluded on this sort of note. My hunch is that when this happens analysis has become a kind of behavior modification: the patient is made aware of and is pushed to renounce his dangerous impulses, but his sense that he is dangerous is never adequately addressed. Renunciation has been facilitated by a reinforcement of the patient's capacity for self-control. The analyst has countertransferentially identified with the patient's harshly critical self, and the patient in turn has reintrojected the analyst's attitude. The patient is then left with the feeling of being "sadder but wiser," able to make himself behave better without ever having the chance to experience fully why he became convinced that he was bad in the first place. The less fortunate of these patients, while symptomatically improved and apparently more successfully adapted, display a kind of resignation and pervasive dysphoria. The more fortunate seek out second analyses.

The Appreciation of Convictions

One of Freud's most powerful statements of the potential and dangers of the transference appears in his postcript to the Dora case. Here he blames the treatment's collapse on his failure to address the transference in a timely and vigorous way:

> I ought to have said to her, "it is from Herr K. that you have made a transference on to me. Have you noticed anything that leads you to suspect me

of evil intentions similar (whether openly or in some sublimated form) to Herr K.'s? Or have you been struck by anything about me or got to know anything about me which has caught your fancy, as happened previously with Herr K.?" (1905b, p. 118).

Dora was treated before Freud fully developed his drive model, before he came to believe that the patient's experience of the analyst was determined by the transference of impulse. It is unlikely that later on he would have asked his patients whether they noticed anything about him that gave them a particular impression. Certainly contemporary drive theorists do not raise such questions. Arlow, for example, suggests that the analyst's "real behavior" is a minor precipitant of tranference impulses, comparable in importance to the day residue that triggers the dream (1985a). Freud's question, on this view, would collude with the patient's own interest in remaining with his preconscious (perceptual) experience.

A vision of transference based on appreciation of the patient's convictions about the analyst returns us to the wisdom of Freud's early advice. I am not, in this connection, suggesting that it is helpful either to confirm or to dispute any convictions the patient might express. At this phase of the work, the analyst must follow the often more difficult path of maintaining an openness to the patient's impressions and an awareness of their plausibility, even when doing so gets uncomfortable. In this respect I am in full agreement with Gill's technical suggestions concerning the analysis of transference. Failing to raise any question about the patient's perceptions forecloses the possibility of exploring the underlying convictions. It also protects the analyst from any distressing thoughts about whether the patient is getting close to something.

Consider the case I supervised in which the analyst focused exclusively on the murderous elements of his patient's dreams. Had the analyst asked "Have you noticed anything in me that you take as a sign of my vulnerability to your ambition or success?" the patient might have been able to address not only his impulses and their history but also his fears and inhibitions. Again, the analyst would have been put in a dangerous position: recall that, from my perspective as his supervisor, he was indeed quite concerned about being outdone by the patient. My line of questioning and interpretation would have made him anxious. It is in the recognition of vulnerability and anxiety that the working through of countertransference occurs, and the analyst's openness to these reactions is the best guar-

antee that all facets of the patient's experience will get adequate attention. Only then will the outcome of treatment be genuinely analytic.

When Freud discussed what he might have done with Dora, he did not suggest stopping with her thoughts about him. Had he inquired about those thoughts, however:

> Her attention would . . . have been turned to some detail in our relations, or in my person or circumstances, behind which there lay concealed something analogous but immeasurably more important concerning Herr K. And when this transference had been cleared up, the analysis would have obtained more access to new memories" (pp. 118–119).

Far from arresting the analytic process, as Arlow claims it would, the analyst's openness to his patient's beliefs about him is precisely the route to a deepened experience. Convictions, like the representations from which they derive, are determined in many ways. Once the convictions are expressed, their various elements—wishes as well as impressions—will be more accessible.

I will conclude with an example of how this can work. A man I had been seeing in therapy for about two years had, with great consistency, maintained a particular set of ideas about me. First he believed that I lead a kind of idyllic personal, emotional, and intellectual life—exactly the sort he would aspire to. Then he felt that with him I was distant, certainly benign but without much interest in him. He reported the following dream: He arrives for a session and notices for the first time that my office is attached to my apartment. The apartment is open to view and he sees that, in contrast to the office, it is quite a mess. The session begins, and I am acting quite in contrast to my usual manner. I am warmer, more intimate, open to talking with him about things that interest us both. We agree enthusiastically about some things and spar combatively about others. He senses in the dream that this is an unusual way for me to act with patients, and he is left with the feeling that he is special to me. The patient, a man with considerable psychological sophistication and some knowledge of psychoanalytic theory, had a quick explanation for the dream. It represents, of course, a wish. He wishes that he had access to the less "perfect" aspects of my life. If he did, he could feel more related to me, more engaged, closer, and that would be very exciting. He reported the dream near the end of a session, and matters rested there.

I was left with a slightly uncomfortable feeling. First, the analysis of the

dream seemed far too glib and too much like what he already was comfortable saying about himself. Second, my office at the time consisted of three rooms—a consulting room, a waiting room, and a rear storage room that was visible from the waiting room. The consulting room was neat and comfortable, the other two were in some disrepair—I had been intending to get them fixed up and they were something of an embarrassment to me. So in the next session I mentioned that perhaps the dream reflected what he had seen. He responded that yes, he had noticed, had even thought about the condition of the outer rooms as he was driving to his session—but what difference did it make? In any case, wasn't that just the day residue, a superficial trigger for an underlying wish?

I said that I wondered: he seemed rather more comfortable with the wish than with the perception. What had he thought about the messiness? There was a silence, and the patient acknowledged that he had felt he had a special understanding of my messiness. He cherished his perception as embodying a chink in my armor, and that the messiness connected us as men. He felt particularly close to me because of this and was excited by his secret knowledge. It was like wrestling, with all the physical contact, sharing, competitiveness, and sexuality involved in tumbling around together.

What I want to emphasize is that by focusing on his disavowed perception, we were able to shift his awareness from the excitement as something wished for to excitement as something actually felt. Needless to say, the analysis does not stop at articulating the perceptions themselves—that would indeed be superficial. But without acknowledging what had been seen, it would not have been possible for this patient fully to experience his elaboration of it: he would have been left with a sense of himself as excited alone, and ultimately as excluded and deprived. In his life history this served not only to protect him from the anxiety generated by his own excitement, but also to protect those around him from awareness of his impact and of their own vulnerability. He invited me to repeat this in the transference, in the service of avoiding anxiety over the condition of my office.

HANS LOEWALD wrote poignantly about the intricate connection between perceptual reality, archaic memory, and passion: "there is neither such a thing as reality nor a real relationship without transference. Any 'real relationship' involves transfer of unconscious images to present-day objects. In fact, present-day objects are objects, and thus real, in the full sense of

the word only to the extent to which this transference . . . is realized" (1960, p. 254).

Transference is anchored in the real, and we become real to our patients through their transference. As we are created in each new analysis, so we are also exposed. We are privileged to witness, as part of our daily work, the dynamic interplay of need and fear, of history and conviction in the origin of experience. But the analytic process will remain vital only if we battle the inescapable temptation to withdraw self-protectively from the unique, often troubling transferences that make us come alive to our patients. Psychoanalytic theory comes to the aid of practice when it affirms both the struggles we all go through to construct our personal worlds and the unique creation represented by each individual human life.

References

Abraham, K. 1924. A short study of the development of the libido, viewed in the light of mental disorders. In *Selected papers of Karl Abraham*. London: Hogarth Press, 1968, pp. 418–501.

Ansbacher, H., and Ansbacher, R. 1956. *The individual psychology of Alfred Adler: a systematic presentation in selections from his writings*. New York: Basic Books.

Apfelbaum, B. 1962. Some problems in contemporary ego psychology. *Journal of the American Psychoanalytic Association*, 10:526–537.

——— 1965. Ego psychology, psychic energy, and the hazards of quantitative explanation in psycho-analytic theory. *International Journal of Psycho-analysis*, 46:168–182.

——— 1966. On ego psychology: a critique of the structural approach to psycho-analytic theory. *International Journal of Psycho-analysis*, 47:451–475.

Arlow, J. 1980. Object concept and object choice. *Psychoanalytic Quarterly*, 49:109–133.

——— 1985a. The concept of psychic reality and other problems. *Journal of the American Psychoanalytic Association*, 33:521–535.

——— 1985b. The structural hypothesis. *In Models of the mind*, ed. A. Rothstein. Workshop series of the American Psychoanalytic Association, monograph 1. New York: International Universities Press, pp. 21–33.

——— and C. Brenner. 1964. *Psychoanalytic concepts and the structural theory*. New York: International Universities Press.

Bacal, H. 1990. Does an object relations theory exist in self psychology? *Psychoanalytic Inquiry*, 10:197–220.

Basch, M. 1987. The interpersonal and the intrapsychic: conflict or harmony? *Contemporary Psychoanalysis*, 23:367–381.

Beebe, B., and F. Lachmann. 1988a. Mother-infant mutual influences and precursors of psychic structure. In *Frontiers of self psychology: progress in self psychology*, vol. 3, ed. A. Goldberg. Hillsdale: Analytic Press, pp. 3–26.

Beebe, B., and F. Lachmann. 1988b. The contribution of mother-infant mutual influence to the origins of self- and object representations. *Psychoanalytic Psychology*, 5:305–357.

Benedek, T. 1949. Dynamics of the countertransference. In *Psychoanalytic investigations: selected papers*. New York: Quadrangle, 1973, pp. 492–499.

Bernfeld, S. 1944. Freud's earliest theories and the school of Helmholtz. *Psychoanalytic Quarterly*, 13:341–362.

Bibring, E. 1936. The development and problems of the theory of instincts. *International Journal of Psycho-analysis*, 22:102–131, 1941.

Bloom, H. 1973. *The anxiety of influence*. New York: Oxford University Press.

Black, M. 1967. Review of A. R. Louch's *Explanation and human action*. *American Journal of Psychology*, 80:655–656.

Boesky, D. 1988. The concept of psychic structure. *Journal of the American Psychoanalytic Association*, 36(suppl):113–135.

Bowlby, J. 1969. *Attachment*. New York: Basic Books.

—— 1973. *Separation: anxiety and anger*. New York: Basic Books.

Brenner, C. 1955. *An elementary textbook of psychoanalysis*. Garden City: Doubleday Anchor Books.

—— 1980a. Metapsychology and psychoanalytic theory. *Psychoanalytic Quarterly*, 49:189–214.

—— 1980b. The psychoanalytic theory of the drives. *Psychoanalytic Quarterly*, 51:171–173.

—— 1982. *The mind in conflict*. New York: International Universities Press.

Breuer, J., and S. Freud. 1895. *Studies on hysteria*. In *The standard edition of the complete psychological works of Sigmund Freud*, vol. 2. London: Hogarth Press.

Bühler, K. 1918. *Die geistige entwicklung des kindes*. Jena: Fischer, 4th ed., 1924.

Compton, A. 1983. The current status of the psychoanalytic theory of instinctual drives, I: drive concept, classification, and development. *Psychoanalytic Quarterly*, 52:364–401.

Curtis, H. 1985. Clinical perspectives on self psychology. *Psychoanalytic Quarterly*, 54:339–378.

Dilman, I. 1983. *Freud and human nature*. Oxford: Blackwell.

Dorpat, T. 1985. *Denial and defense in the therapeutic situation*. New York: Aronson.

Eagle, M. 1980. A critical examination of motivational explanation in psychoanalysis. In *Mind and medicine: explanation and evaluation in psychiatry and medicine*, ed. L. Laudan. Berkeley: University of California Press, 1983, pp. 311–353.

—— 1984. *Recent developments in psychoanalysis: a critical evaluation*. New York: McGraw-Hill.

—— 1987. The psychoanalytic and the cognitive unconscious. In *Theories of the unconscious and theories of the self*, ed. R. Stern. Hillsdale: Analytic Press, pp. 155–189.

Edelson, M. 1984. *Hypothesis and evidence in psychoanalysis*. Chicago: University of Chicago Press.

Erikson, E. 1943. Observations on the Yurok: childhood and world image. *University of California Publications in American Archeology and Ethology*, 35:257–301.

——— 1962. Reality and actuality. *Journal of the American Psychoanalytic Association*, 10:451–474.

——— 1963. *Childhood and society*, 2nd ed. New York: Norton.

Fairbairn, W.R.D. 1940. Schizoid factors in the personality. In *An object-relations theory of the personality*. New York: Basic Books, 1952, pp. 3–27. *(ORT)*.

——— 1941. A revised psychopathology of the psychoses and psychoneuroses. *ORT*, pp. 28–58.

——— 1943. Repression and the return of bad objects (with special reference to the "war neuroses"). *ORT*, pp. 59–81.

——— 1944. Endopsychic structure considered in terms of object-relationships. *ORT*, pp. 82–132.

——— 1946. Object-relationships and dynamic structure. *ORT*, pp. 137–151.

——— 1951. Addendum to endopsychic structure considered in terms of object-relationships. *ORT*, pp. 133–136.

——— 1952. *Psychoanalytic studies of the personality*. London: Routledge and Kegan Paul.

——— 1958. On the nature and aims of psycho-analytical treatment. *International Journal of Psycho-analysis*, 39:374–385.

Fenichel, O. 1935. A critique of the death instinct. In *The collected papers of Otto Fenichel*, 1st series. New York: Norton, 1953, pp. 363–372.

——— 1941. *Problems of psychoanalytic technique*. New York: Psychoanalytic Quarterly.

——— 1945. *The psychoanalytic theory of neurosis*. New York: Norton.

Fisher, C. 1965. Psychoanalytic implications of recent research on sleep and dreaming. *Journal of the American Psychoanalytic Association*, 13:197–303.

Fisher, S., and R. Greenberg. 1978. *The scientific evaluation of Freud's theories and therapy*. New York: Basic Books.

Fodor, J. 1981. *Representations: philosophical essays on the foundations of cognitive science*. Cambridge: MIT Press.

Freud, A. 1936. *The ego and the mechanisms of defense*. New York: International Universities Press.

Freud, S. *On aphasia*. New York: International Universities Press, 1953. Subsequent Freud citations are from *The standard edition of the complete psychological works of Sigmund Freud*, vols. 1–24, ed. J. Strachey. London: Hogarth Press, 1953–1974. *(SE)*.

——— 1895. *Project for a scientific psychology. SE*, 1:281–397.

——— 1894. The neuro-psychoses of defense. *SE*, 3:43–68.

——— 1896a. Heredity and the aetiology of neuroses. *SE*, 3:141–156.

Freud, S. 1896b. Further remarks on the neuro-psychoses of defense. *SE,* 3:159–185.

—— 1896c. The aetiology of hysteria. *SE,* 3:189–221.

—— 1898. Sexuality in the aetiology of the neuroses. *SE,* 3:261–285.

—— 1899. Screen memories. *SE,* 3:301–322.

—— 1900. *The interpretation of dreams. SE,* 4, 5.

—— 1901. *The psychopathology of everyday life. SE,* 6.

—— 1905a. *Three essays on the theory of sexuality. SE,* 7:125–245.

—— 1905b. *Fragment of an analysis of a case of hysteria. SE,* 7:1–122.

—— 1905c. *Jokes and their relation to the unconscious. SE,* 8.

—— 1906. My views on the part played by sexuality in the aetiology of the neuroses. *SE,* 7:269–279.

—— 1907. Delusions and dreams in Jensen's Gradiva. *SE,* 9:1–95.

—— 1909. Analysis of a phobia in a five-year-old boy. *SE,* 10:1–149.

—— 1910a. Leonardo da Vinci and a memory of his childhood. *SE,* 11:57–137.

—— 1910b. Five lectures on psycho-analysis. *SE,* 11:7–55.

—— 1910c. The psycho-analytic view of psychogenic disturbance of vision. *SE,* 11:209–218.

—— 1911a. Formulations on the two principles of mental functioning. *SE,* 12:218–226.

—— 1911b. Psycho-analytic notes on an autobiographical account of a case of paranoia (dementia paranoides). *SE,* 12:1–82.

—— 1912a. The dynamics of transference. *SE,* 12:97–108.

—— 1912b. On the universal tendency to debasement in the sphere of love. *SE,* 11:177–190.

—— 1912–13. *Totem and taboo. SE,* 13:1–162.

—— 1913. On beginning the treatment (further recommendations on the technique of psycho-analysis, I). *SE,* 12:121–144.

—— 1914a. On narcissism: an introduction. *SE,* 14:67–102.

—— 1914b. On the history of the psycho-analytic movement. *SE,* 14:1–66.

—— 1914c. Remembering, repeating and working-through (further recommendations on the technique of psycho-analysis, II). *SE,* 12:145–156.

—— 1915a. Instincts and their vicissitudes. *SE,* 14:117–140.

—— 1915b. Repression. *SE,* 14:141–158.

—— 1915c. The unconscious. *SE,* 14:159–215.

—— 1915d. Observations on transference love (further recommendations on the technique of psycho-analysis, III). *SE,* 12:157–171.

—— 1916–17. *Introductory lectures on psycho-analysis. SE,* 15, 16.

—— 1917a. Mourning and melancholia. *SE,* 14:237–258.

—— 1917b. A metapsychological supplement to the theory of dreams. *SE,* 14:217–235.

—— 1918. From the history of an infantile neurosis. *SE,* 17:3–122.

—— 1919. 'A child is being beaten,' a contribution to the study of the origin of sexual perversions. *SE*, 17:175–204.

—— 1920. *Beyond the pleasure principle. SE*, 18:3–64.

—— 1921. Group psychology and the analysis of the ego. *SE*, 18:65–143.

—— 1923a. *The ego and the id. SE*, 19:1–66.

—— 1923b. Two enclyclopedia artices. *SE*, 18:233–259.

—— 1925a. Some additional notes on dream-interpretation as a whole. *SE*, 19:125–138.

—— 1925b. An autobiographical study. *SE*, 20:1–74.

—— 1926. *Inhibitions, symptoms and anxiety. SE*, 20:75–175.

—— 1927. *The future of an illusion. SE*, 21:1–56.

—— 1928. Appendix to Doestoevski and parricide. *SE*, 21:195–196.

—— 1930. *Civilization and its discontents. SE*, 21:59–145.

—— 1931. Libidinal types. *SE*, 21:215–220.

—— 1933. *New introductory lectures on pscyho-analysis. SE*, 22:1–182.

—— 1940. *An outline of psycho-analysis. SE*, 23:139–207.

—— 1950. Extracts from the Fliess papers. *SE*, 1:173–280.

—— 1987 [1915]. Overview of the transference neuroses. In *A phylogenetic fantasy*, ed. I. Grubrich-Simitis. Cambridge: Harvard University Press.

Friedman, J., and J. Alexander. 1983. Psychoanalysis and natural science: Freud's 1895 Project revisited. *International Review of Psychoanalysis*, 10:303–318.

Friedman, L. 1980. Kohut: a book review essay. *Psychoanalytic Quarterly*, 49:393–422. In *The anatomy of psychotherapy*. Hillsdale: Analytic Press, 1988, pp. 368–388.

Friedman, M. 1985. Toward a reconceptualization of guilt. *Contemporary Psychoanalysis*, 21:501–547.

Fromm, E. 1941. *Escape from freedom*. New York: Avon.

Gay, P. 1985. *Freud for historians*. New York: Oxford University Press.

—— 1988. *Freud: a life for our time*. New York: Norton.

Gedo, J. 1979. *Beyond interpretation*. New York: International Universities Press.

Gill, M. 1963. *Topography and systems in psychoanalytic theory. Psychological Issues*, monograph 10. New York: International Universities Press.

—— 1976. Metapsychology is not psychology. In *Psychology versus metapsychology: psychoanalytic essays in memory of George S. Klein*, ed. M. Gill and P. Holzman. *Psychological Issues*, monograph 36. New York: International Universities Press.

—— 1982. *Analysis of transference*, vol. 1. New York: International Universities Press.

—— 1983a. The point of view of psychoanalysis: energy discharge or person. *Psychoanalysis and Contemporary Thought*, 6:523–551.

—— 1983b. The interpersonal paradigm and the degree of the therapist's involvement. *Contemporary Psychoanalysis*, 19:200–237.

—— 1987. The analyst as participant. *Psychoanalytic Inquiry*, 7:249–259.

Gill, M., and G. Klein. 1964. The structuring of drive and reality: David Rapaport's contributions to psychoanalysis and psychology. In *The collected papers of David Rapaport*, ed. M. Gill. New York: Basic Books, 1967, pp. 8–34.

Glover, E. 1955. *The technique of psycho-analysis*. New York: International Universities Press.

Goldberg, A. 1988. *A fresh look at psychoanalysis: the view from self psychology*. Hillsdale: Analytic Press.

Greenberg, J. 1981. Prescription or description: the therapeutic action of psychoanalysis. *Contemporary Psychoanalysis*, 17:239–257.

——— 1986. Heinz Hartmann and drive theory: toward a re-evaluation. *Psychoanalytic Inquiry*, 6:523–541.

——— and S. Mitchell. 1983. *Object relations in psychoanalytic theory*. Cambridge: Harvard University Press.

Greenson, R. 1967. *The technique and practice of psychoanalysis*, vol. 1. New York: International Universities Press.

Grünbaum, A. 1984. *The foundations of psychoanalysis*. Berkeley: University of California Press.

Groos, K. 1901. *The play of man*. New York: Appleton.

Hartmann, H. 1939a. *Ego psychology and the problem of adaptation*. New York: International Universities Press.

——— 1939b. Psychoanalysis and the concept of health. In *Essays on ego psychology*. New York: International Universities Press, pp. 1–18. *(EEP)*.

——— 1948. Comments on the psychoanalytic theory of instinctual drives. *EEP*, pp. 69–89.

——— 1950. Comments on the psychoanalytic theory of the ego. *EEP*, pp. 113–141.

——— 1951. Technical implications of ego psychology. *EEP*, pp. 142–154.

——— 1952. The mutual influences in the development of ego and id. *EEP*, pp. 155–181.

——— 1953. Contribution to the metapsychology of schizophrenia. *EEP*, pp. 182–206.

——— 1955. Notes on the theory of sublimation. *EEP*, pp. 215–240.

——— 1956. Notes on the reality principle. *EEP*, pp. 241–267.

——— 1960. *Psychoanalysis and moral values*. New York: International Universities Press.

——— and E. Kris. 1945. The genetic approach in psychoanalysis. In *Papers on psychoanalytic psychology. Psychological Issues*, monograph 14. New York: International Universities Press, pp. 7–26. *(PPP)*.

——— ——— and R. Loewenstein. 1946. Comments on the formation of psychic structure. *PPP*, pp. 27–55.

——— ——— and ——— 1949. Notes on the theory of aggression. *PPP*, pp. 56–85.

——— ——— and ——— 1953. The function of theory in psychoanalysis. *PPP*, pp. 117–143.

Hartmann, H., and R. Loewenstein. 1962. Notes on the superego. *PPP*, pp. 144–181.

Hendrick, I. 1942. Instinct and the ego during infancy. *Psychoanalytic Quarterly*, 11:33–58.

——— 1943. The discussion of the 'instinct to master.' *Psychoanalytic Quarterly*, 12:561–565.

Hoffman, I. 1983. The patient as interpreter of the analyst's experience. *Contemporary Psychoanalysis*, 19:389–422.

Holt, R. 1962. A critical examination of Freud's concept of bound vs. free cathexis. *Journal of the American Psychoanalytic Association*, 10:475–525.

——— 1965a. Ego autonomy re-evaluated. *International Journal of Psychiatry*, 3:481–503, 1967.

——— 1965b. A review of some of Freud's biological assumptions and their influence on his theories. In *Psychoanalysis and current biological thought*, ed. N. Greenfield and W. Lewis. Madison: University of Wisconsin Press, pp. 93–124.

——— 1967a. Beyond vitalism and mechanism: Freud's concept of psychic energy. In *Science and psychoanalysis*, vol. 11, ed. J. Masserman. New York: Grune and Stratton, pp. 1–41.

——— 1967b. Editors' footnote in G. Klein, Peremptory ideation: structure and force in motivated ideas. In *Motives and thought: psychoanalytic essays in honor of David Rapaport*, ed. R. Holt. *Psychological Issues*, monograph 18/19. New York: International Universities Press, pp. 78–128.

——— 1967c. On freedom, autonomy, and the redirection of psychoanalytic theory: a rejoinder. *International Journal of Psychiatry*, 3:524–536.

——— 1975. The past and future of ego psychology. *Psychoanalytic Quarterly*, 44:550–576.

——— 1976. Drive or wish? A reconsideration of the psychoanalytic theory of motivation. In *Psychology versus metapsychology: psychoanalytic essays in memory of George S. Klein*, ed. M. Gill and P. Holzman. *Psychological Issues*, monograph 36. New York: International Universities Press, pp. 158–197.

——— 1981. The death and transfiguration of metapsychology. *International Review of Psycho-analysis*, 8:129–143.

——— 1985. The current status of psychoanalytic theory. *Psychoanalytic Psychology*, 2:289–315.

Isaacs, S. 1943. The nature and function of phantasy. In M. Klein, P. Heimann, S. Isaacs, and J. Riviere, *Developments in psycho-analysis*. London: Hogarth Press, 1952.

Jacobson, E. 1954. The self and the object world. *Psychoanalytic Study of the Child*, 9:75–127.

——— 1964. *The self and the object world*. New York: International Universities Press.

Joffe, W., and J. Sandler. 1968. Adaptation, affects, and the representational world. In *From safety to superego*. New York: Guilford, pp. 221–234.

Jung, C. 1913. The theory of psychoanalysis. In *Critique of psychoanalysis*. Princeton: Princton University Press, 1961, pp. 1–144.

Kanzer, M. 1973. Two prevalent misconceptions about Freud's "Project" (1895). *Annual of Psychoanalysis*, 1:88–103.

—— 1983. The inconstant 'principle of constancy.' *Journal of the American Psychoanalytic Association*, 31:843–865.

Kernberg, O. 1976. *Object relations theory and clinical psychoanalysis*. New York: Aronson.

—— 1980. *Internal world and external reality*. New York: Aronson.

—— 1982. Self, ego, affects, and drives. *Journal of the American Psychoanalytic Association*, 30:893–917.

—— 1987. Projection and projective identification: developmental and clinical aspects. In *Projection, identification, projective identification*, ed. J. Sandler. New York: International Universities Press, pp. 93–115.

Khan, M. 1960. Regression and integration in the analytic setting: a clinical essay on the transference and counter-transference aspects of these phenomena. In *The privacy of the self*. New York: International Universities Press, 1974, pp. 136–167.

Klauber, J. 1968. On the dual use of historical and scientific method in psychoanalysis. In *Difficulties in the analytic encounter*. New York: Aronson, 1981, pp. 181–204.

Klein, G. 1967. Peremptory ideation: structure and force in motivated ideas. In *Motives and thought: psychoanalytic essays in honor of David Rapaport*, ed. R. Holt. *Psychological Issues*, monograph 18/19. New York: International Universities Press, pp. 78–128.

—— 1976. *Psychoanalytic theory: an exploration of essentials*. New York: International Universities Press.

Klein, M. 1932. *The psycho-analysis of children*. London: Hogarth Press.

Klein, Mi., and D. Tribich. 1981. Kernberg's object-relations theory: a critical evaluation. *International Journal of Psycho-analysis*, 62:27–43.

Kohut, H. 1971. *The analysis of the self*. New York: International Universities Press.

—— 1975. On female sexuality. In *The search for the self: selected writings of Heinz Kohut, 1950–1978*, ed. P. Ornstein. New York: International Universities Press, 1978, pp. 783–792.

—— 1977. *The restoration of the self*. New York: International Universities Press.

—— 1979. The two analyses of Mr. Z. *International Journal of Psycho-analysis*, 60:3–27.

—— 1980. Two letters: from a letter to one of the participants at the Chicago conference on the psychology of the self; from a letter to a colleague. In *Advances in self psychology*, ed. A. Goldberg. New York: International Universities Press, pp. 449–472.

—— 1982. Introspection, empathy, and the semi-circle of mental health. *International Journal of Psycho-analysis*, 63:395–405.

—— 1984. *How does analysis cure?* Chicago: University of Chicago Press.

Kris, A. 1977. Either-or dilemmas. *Psychoanalytic Study of the Child*, 32:91–117.

—— 1984. The conflicts of ambivalence. *Psychoanalytic Study of the Child*, 39:213–234.

Kris, E. 1947. The nature of psychoanalytic propositions and their validation. In *The selected papers of Ernst Kris*. New Haven: Yale University Press, 1975, pp. 3–23.

—— 1955. Neutralization and sublimation: observations on young children. *Psychoanalytic Study of the Child*, 10:30–46.

—— 1956. On some vicissitudes of insight in psychoanalysis. In *The selected papers*. New Haven: Yale University Press, 1975, pp. 252–271.

Krüll, M. 1986. *Freud and his father*. New York: Norton.

Kubie, L. 1947. The fallacious use of quantitative concepts in dynamic psychology. *Psychoanalytic Quarterly*, 16:507–518.

Lachmann, F. 1986. Interpretation of psychic conflict and adversarial relationships: a self-psychological perspective. *Psychoanalytic Psychology*, 3:341–355.

Lampl-de Groot, J. 1956. The theory of instinctual drives. *International Journal of Psycho-analysis*, 37:354–359.

LaPlanche, J., and J-B. Pontalis. 1973. *The language of psycho-analysis*, tr. D. Nicholson-Smith. New York: Norton.

Levenson, E. 1972. *The fallacy of understanding*. New York: Basic Books.

—— 1985. The interpersonal (Sullivanian) model. In *Models of the mind: their relationships to clinical work*, ed. A. Rothstein. New York: International Universities Press, pp. 49–67.

—— 1987. An interpersonal perspective. *Psychoanalytic Inquiry*, 7:207–214.

Lichtenberg, J. 1983a. *Psychoanalysis and infant research*. Hillsdale: Analytic Press.

—— 1983b. Is there a weltanschauung to be developed from psychoanalysis? In *The future of psychoanalysis*, ed. A. Goldberg. New York: International Universities Press, pp. 203–238.

—— 1988. A theory of motivational-functional systems as psychic structures. *Journal of the American Psychoanalytic Association*, 36(suppl):57–72.

—— 1989. *Psychoanalysis and motivation*. Hillsdale, NJ: Analytic Press.

Loewald, H. 1960. On the therapeutic action of psychoanalysis. In *Papers on psychoanalysis*. New Haven: Yale University Press, 1980, pp. 221–256. *(PP)*.

—— 1969. Freud's conception of the negative therapeutic reaction, with comments on instinct theory. *PP*, pp. 315–325.

—— 1970. Psychoanalytic theory and the psychoanalytic process. *PP*, pp. 277–301.

—— 1971. On motivation and instinct theory. *PP*, pp. 102–137.

—— 1977. Instinct theory, object relations, and psychic structure formation. *PP*, pp. 207–218.

—— 1979. The waning of the Oedipus complex. *Journal of the American Psychoanalytic Association*, 27:751–775.

Loewenstein, R. 1940. The vital or somatic instincts. *International Journal of Psycho-analysis,* 21:377–400.

—— 1965. Observational data and theory in psychoanalysis. In *Drives, affects, behavior,* vol. 2, ed. M. Schur. New York: International Universities Press, pp. 38–59.

Lustman, S. 1968. The economic point of view and defence. *Psychoanalytic Study of the Child,* 23:189–203.

Mahler, M. 1946. Ego psychology applied to behavior problems. In *Modern trends in child psychiatry,* ed. N.D.C. Lewis and B. L. Pacella. New York: International Universities Press.

—— 1968. *On human symbiosis and the vicissitudes of individuation,* vol. 1, *Infantile psychosis.* New York: International Universities Press.

—— and B. Gosliner. 1955. On symbiotic child psychosis: genetic, dynamic and restitutive aspects. *Psychoanalytic Study of the Child,* 10:195–212.

—— F. Pine, and A. Bergman. 1975. *The psychological birth of the human infant: symbiosis and individuation.* New York: Basic Books.

Mancia, M. 1983. Archaelogy of Freudian thought and the history of neurophysiology. *International Review of Psycho-analysis,* 10:185–192.

McGuire, W. 1974. *The Freud/Jung letters.* Princeton: Princeton University Press.

Mitchell, S. 1981. Twilight of the idols. *Contemporary Psychoanalysis,* 17:374–398.

—— 1984. Object relations theories and the developmental tilt. *Contemporary Psychoanalysis,* 20:473–499.

—— 1988. *Relational concepts in psychoanalysis: an integration.* Cambridge: Harvard University Press.

Mittelman, B. 1954. Motility in infants, children, and adults. *Psychoanalytic Study of the Child,* 9:142–177.

Modell, A. 1990. Some notes on object relations, "classical" theory and the problems of instincts (drives). *Psychoanalytic Inquiry,* 10:182–196.

Money, J., and A. Ehrhardt. 1972. *Man and woman, boy and girl.* Baltimore: Johns Hopkins University Press.

Moore, B., and B. Fine, eds. 1990. *Psychoanalytic terms and concepts.* New Haven: American Psychoanalytic Association and Yale University Press.

Myerson, P. 1981a. The nature of the transactions that enhance the progressive phases of psychoanalysis. *International Journal of Psycho-analysis,* 62:91–103.

—— 1981b. The nature of the transactions that occur in other than classical analysis. *International Review of Psycho-analysis,* 8:173–189.

Nacht, S. 1952. The mutual influences in the development of ego and id. *Psychoanalytic Study of the Child,* 7:54–59.

Nilsson, L. 1990. *A child is born.* New York: Delacorte Press/Seymour Lawrence.

Novey, S. 1957. A re-evaluation of certain aspects of the theory of instinctual drives in the light of modern ego psychology. *International Journal of Psycho-analysis,* 38:137–145.

Nunberg, H. 1930. The synthetic function of the ego. In *Practice and theory of psychoanalysis.* New York: International Universities Press, 1960, pp. 120–136.

Ogden, T. 1984. Instinct, phantasy, and psychological deep structure. *Contemporary Psychoanalysis*, 20:500–525.

———— 1989. *The primitive edge of experience*. New York: Aronson.

Ornstein, P. 1978. The evolution of Heinz Kohut's psychoanalytic psychology of the self. In *The search for the self: selected writings of Heinz Kohut, 1950–1978*, ed. P. Ornstein. New York: International Universities Press, 1978, pp. 1–106.

Ortega y Gasset, J. 1941. History as a system. In *History as a system and other essays toward a philosophy of history*. New York: Norton, pp. 165–233.

Panel, H. Dahl, reporter. 1968. Psychoanalytic theory of the instinctual drives in relation to recent developments. *Journal of the American Psychoanalytic Association*, 16:613–637.

Panel, R. Lieder, reporter. 1984. The neutrality of the analyst in the analytic situation. *Journal of the American Psychoanalytic Association*, 32:573–585.

Parisi, T. 1987. Why Freud failed: some implications for neurophysiology and sociobiology. *American Psychologist*, 42:235–245.

Pine, F. 1985. *Developmental theory and clinical process*. New Haven: Yale University Press.

———— 1988. Motivation, personality organization, and the four psychologies of psychoanalysis. *Journal of the American Psychoanalytic Association*, 37:31–64.

Plaut, E. 1984. Ego instincts: a concept whose time has come. *Psychoanalytic Study of the Child*, 39:235–258.

Poland, W. 1984. On the analyst's neutrality. *Journal of the American Psychoanalytic Association*, 32:283–299.

Pulver, S. 1988 Psychic structure, function, process, and content: toward a definition. *Journal of the American Psychoanalytic Association*, 36(suppl):165–189.

Rangell, L. 1954. Similarities and differences between psychoanalysis and dynamic psychotherapy. *Journal of the American Psychoanalytic Association*, 2:734–744.

———— 1982. The self in psychoanalytic theory. *Journal of the American Psychoanalytic Assocation*, 30:863–891.

Rapaport, D. 1947. Dynamic psychology and Kantian epistemology. In *The collected papers of David Rapaport*, ed. M. Gill. New York: Basic Books, 1967, pp. 289–298. *(CP)*.

———— 1951. The autonomy of the ego. *CP*, pp. 357–367.

———— 1957. The theory of ego autonomy: a generalization. *CP*, pp. 722–744.

———— 1958. A historical survey of psychoanalytic ego psychology. *CP*, pp. 745–757.

———— 1959. *The structure of psychoanalytic theory: a systematizing attempt*. *Psychological Issues*, monograph 6. New York: International Universities Press, 1960.

———— 1960. On the psychoanalytic theory of motivation. *CP*, pp. 853–915.

———— 1967. A theoretical analysis of the superego concept. *CP*, pp. 685–709.

Rapaport, D., and M. Gill. 1959. The points of view and assumptions of metapsychology. *CP*, pp. 795–811.

Reiser, M. 1985. Converging sectors of psychoanalysis and neurobiology: mutual challenges and opportunity. *Journal of the American Psychoanalytic Association,* 33:11–34.

Rubinstein, B. 1967. Explanation and mere description: a metascientific examination of certain aspects of the psychoanalytic theory of motivation. In *Motives and thought: psychoanalytic essays in honor of David Rapaport,* ed. R. Holt. *Psychological Issues,* monograph 18/19. New York: International Universities Press, pp. 20–77.

———— 1976. On the possibility of a strictly clinical psychoanalytic theory: an essay in the philosophy of psychoanalysis. In *Psychology versus metapsychology: psychoanalytic essays in memory of George S. Klein,* ed. M. Gill and P. Holzman. *Psychological Issues,* Monograph 36. New York: International Universities Press, pp. 229–264.

Rugh, R., and L. Shettles. 1971. *From conception to birth: the drama of life's beginnings.* New York: Harper and Row.

Sandler, J. 1962. Psychology and psychoanalysis. In *From safety to superego.* New York: Guilford, pp. 45–57. *(SS).*

———— 1972. The role of affects in psychoanalytic theory. *SS,* pp. 285–297.

———— 1974. Psychological conflict and the structural model: some clinical and theoretical implications. *International Journal of Psycho-analysis,* 55:53–62.

———— 1981. Unconscious wishes and human relationships. *Contemporary Psychoanalysis,* 17:180–196.

———— 1983. Reflections on some relations between psychoanalytic concepts and psychoanalytic practice. *International Journal of Psycho-analysis,* 64:35–45.

———— C. Dare, and A. Holder. 1973. *The patient and the analyst: the basis of the psychoanalytic process.* London: Maresfield Reprints, 1979.

———— and W. Joffe. 1965. Obsessional manifestations in children. *SS,* pp. 142–153).

———— and ———— 1966. On sublimation. *SS,* pp. 191–207.

———— and ———— 1968. Psychoanalytic psychology and learning theory. *SS,* pp. 255–263.

———— and ———— 1969. Toward a basic psychoanalytic model. *SS,* pp. 235–254).

———— and B. Rosenblatt. 1962. The concept of the representational world. *Psychoanalytic Study of the Child,* 17:128–145.

———— and A. Sandler. 1978. On the development of object relationships and affects. *International Journal of Psycho-analysis,* 59:285–296.

———— and ———— 1983. The "second censorship," the "three box model" and some technical implications. *International Journal of Psycho-analysis,* 64:413–425.

———— and ———— 1987. The past unconscious, the present unconscious and the vicissitudes of guilt. *International Journal of Psycho-analysis,* 68:331–341.

Schafer, R. 1968. *Aspects of internalization.* New York: International Universities Press.

———— 1970. The psychoanalytic vision of reality. In *A new language for psychoanalysis*. New Haven: Yale University Press, 1976, pp. 22–56.

———— 1976. *A new language for psychoanalysis*. New Haven: Yale University Press.

———— 1980. *Narrative actions in psychoanalysis*. Worcester: Clark University Press, 1981.

———— 1983. *The analytic attitude*. New York: Basic Books.

———— 1985. The interpretation of psychic reality, developmental influences, and unconscious communication. *Journal of the American Psychoanalytic Association*, 33:537–554.

———— 1988. Discussion of panel presentations on psychic structure. *Journal of the American Psychoanalytic Association*, 36(suppl):295–312.

Schur, M. 1958. The ego and the id in anxiety. *Psychoanalytic Study of the Child*, 13:190–220.

———— 1966. *The id and the regulatory principles of mental functioning*. New York: International Universities Press.

Schwartz, F. 1981. Psychic structure. *International Journal of Psycho-analysis*, 62:61–72.

Schwartz, W. 1984. The two concepts of action and responsibility in psychoanalysis. *Journal of the American Psychoanalytic Association*, 32:557–572.

Silverman, D. 1986. A multi-model approach: looking at clinical data from three theoretical perspectives. *Psychoanalytic Psychology*, 3:121–132.

Silverman, L., F. Lachmann, and R. Milich. 1982. *The search for oneness*. New York: International Universities Press.

Silverman, M. 1987. Clinical material. *Psychoanalytic Inquiry*, 7:147–165.

Slavin, M. 1985. The origins of psychic conflict and the adaptive function of repression: an evolutionary biological view. *Psychoanalysis and Contemporary Thought*, 8:407–440.

Smith, J. 1986. Dualism revisited: Schafer, Hartmann, and Freud. *Psychoanalytic Inquiry*, 6:543–573.

Solms, M., and M. Saling. 1986. On psychoanalysis and neuroscience: Freud's attitude to the localizationist tradition. *International Journal of Psycho-analysis*, 67:397–416.

Spence, D. 1982. *Narrative truth and historical truth*. New York: Norton.

Stern, D. 1985. *The interpersonal world of the infant*. New York: Basic Books.

Stolorow, R., and F. Lachmann. 1980. *Psychoanalysis of developmental arrests*. New York: International Universities Press.

Strachey, J. 1934. The nature of the therapeutic action of psycho-analysis. *International Journal of Psycho-analysis*, 15:127-159.

———— 1957. Editor's note to "Instincts and their vicissitudes." In Freud, *SE*, 14:111–116.

Sullivan, H. S. 1953. *The interpersonal theory of psychiatry*. New York: Norton.

———— 1954. *The psychiatric interview*. New York: Norton.

———— 1964. *The fusion of psychiatry and social science*. New York: Norton.

Sulloway, F. 1979. *Freud: biologist of the mind*. New York: Basic Books.

Thurber, J. 1936. The admiral on the wheel. In *Let your mind alone!* New York: Harper, 1937.

Wachtel, P. 1982. Vicious circles: the self and the rhetoric of emerging and unfolding. *Contemporary Psychoanalysis,* 18:259–273.

Waelder, R. 1930. The principle of multiple function. *Psychoanalytic Quarterly,* 15:45–62, 1936.

—— 1960. *Basic theory of psychoanalysis.* New York: International Universities Press.

—— 1962. Psychoanalysis, scientific method, and philosophy. *Journal of the American Psychoanalytic Association,* 10:617–637.

Wallerstein, R. 1976. Psychoanalysis as a science: its present status and its future tasks. In *Psychology versus metapsychology: psychoanalytic essays in memory of George S. Klein,* ed. M. Gill and P. Holzman. *Psychological Issues,* monograph 36. New York: International Universities Press, pp. 198–228.

Weiss, J., H. Sampson, and the Mount Zion Psychotherapy Research Group. *The psychoanalytic process: theory, clinical observation, and empirical research.* New York: Guilford.

White, R. 1959. Motivation reconsidered: the concept of competence. *Psychological Review,* 66:297–333.

—— 1963. *Ego and reality in psychoanalytic theory. Psychological Issues,* monograph 11. New York: International Universities Press.

Winnicott, D. W. 1954–55. The depressive position in normal emotional development. In *Through paediatrics to psycho-analysis.* London: Hogarth Press, 1958, pp. 262–277.

—— 1958. The capacity to be alone. In *The maturational process and the facilitating environment.* New York: International Universities Press, 1965, pp. 29–36. *(MP).*

—— 1960. Ego distortion in terms of true and false self. *MP,* pp. 140–152.

—— 1962. Ego integration in child development. *MP,* pp. 56–63.

—— 1963. Psychiatric disorder in terms of infantile maturational process. *MP,* pp. 230–241.

Wolf, E. 1980. On the developmental line of selfobject relations. In *Advances in self psychology,* ed. A. Goldberg. New York: International Universities Press, pp. 117–130.

—— 1983. Empathy and countertransference. In *The future of psychoanalysis,* ed. A. Goldberg. New York: International Universities Press, pp. 309–326.

—— 1985. Self psychology and the neuroses. *Annual of Psychoanalysis,* 12/13:57–68.

Index

DATE DUE